Self-assessment for the MRCP Part 2 Written Paper:
Volume 1
Picture Tests

Narinder Bajaj MA MRCP PhD
Honorary Lecturer in Neurology
Specialist Registrar in Neurology
National Hospital for Neurology
London

Balwinder Bajaj BSc MRCP PhD
Consultant Physician and Cardiologist
The Royal Oldham Hospital
Oldham

Karim Meeran MD FRCP
Consultant Endocrinologist
Charing Cross and Hammersmith Hospitals
London

EDITORIAL ADVISOR
Huw Beynon BSc MD FRCP
Consultant Physician and Rheumatologist
The Royal Free Hospital School of Medicine
Royal Free Hospital
London

Blackwell
Science

© 2002 by Blackwell Science Ltd
a Blackwell Publishing company
Editorial Offices:
Osney Mead, Oxford OX2 0EL, UK
  Tel: +44 (0) 1865 206206
108 Cowley Road, Oxford OX4 1JF, UK
  Tel: +44 (0) 1865 791100
Blackwell Publishing USA, 350 Main Street, Malden, MA 02148-5018, USA
  Tel: +1 781 388 8250
Iowa State Press, a Blackwell Publishing Company, 2121 State Avenue, Ames, Iowa 50014-8300, USA
  Tel: +1 515 292 0140
Blackwell Munksgaard, Nørre Søgade 35, PO Box 2148, Copenhagen, DK-1016, Denmark
  Tel: +45 77 33 33 33
Blackwell Publishing Asia, 54 University Street, Carlton, Victoria 3053, Australia
  Tel: +61 (0)3 9347 0300
Blackwell Verlag, Kurfürstendamm 57, 10707 Berlin, Germany
  Tel: +49 (0)30 32 79 060
Blackwell Publishing, 10 rue Casimir Delavigne, 75006 Paris, France
  Tel: +33 1 53 10 33 10

First published 2002

Library of Congress Cataloging-in-Publication Data

Self-assessment for the MRCP part 2 written paper/
  Narinder Bajaj . . . [et al.].
      v. <>   cm.
  Includes index.
  Contents: v. 1   Picture tests.
  ISBN 0-632-06439-0
  1. Internal medicine—Examinations, questions, etc.   I. Bajaj, Narinder.
RC58 .S477   2001
616′.0076—dc21   2001037620

ISBN 0-632-06439-0

A Catalogue record for this title is available from the British Library

Set in 8/10 Frutiger Condensed by Best-set Typesetter Ltd, Hong Kong
Printed and bound in Slovenia by Mladinska knjiga tiskarna d.d.

For further information on Blackwell Science, visit our website:
www.blackwell-science.com

Self-assessment for the MRCP Part 2 Written Paper:
Volume 1 Picture Tests

Contents

Preface

This book is part of a series of three, designed to provide a revision course for the written part of the MRCP examination. Together with Volume 2 (Case Histories) and Volume 3 (Data Interpretation), they comprise a significant volume of work giving ample coverage of the MRCP syllabus.

This volume containing 165 slides, encompasses a wide range of general medical signs and contains many unique examples. We are indebted to Professor Sanjeev Krishna, for the donation of a large portion of this collection.

The writing of this text has been a lengthy one and we would like to thank all members of our respective families for their support and patience during this time. NPSB and BPSB would especially like to thank their father (a long established author) for his words of wisdom.

NPSB, BPSB, KM 2001

Acknowledgements

We would like to acknowledge the contribution of the following to the photographs shown in this book:

Professor Sanjeev Krishna FRCP DPhil
Professor of Molecular Parasitology and Medicine
Department of Infectious Diseases
St George's Hospital
London

Professor T.M.E. Davis FRCAP DPhil
University of Western Australia
Department of Medicine
Fremantle Hospital
Fremantle
Australia

Question 1

This patient presented with dysphagia.

A What study has been performed?

B What abnormality is shown?

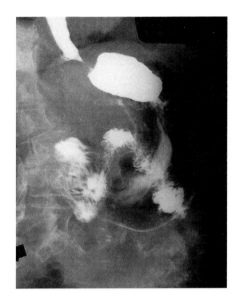

Question 2

A What disorder is shown here?

B Give four conditions associated with this skin appearance.

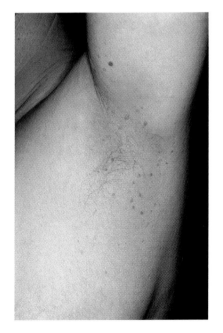

Answer 1

A Barium meal and follow-through.

B 'Apple core' lesion of distal oesophagus, suggestive of carcinoma of the oesophagus.

Answer 2

A Acanthosis nigricans.

B Associations:
visceral malignancy—usually adenocarcinoma,
insulin resistant diabetes mellitus,
acromegaly/Cushing's syndrome/polycystic ovary disease,
Prader–Willi syndrome,
familial.

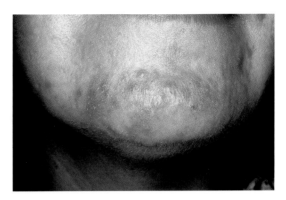

Question 3

A What is this skin lesion?

B Give two complications that may occur.

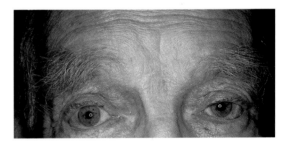

Question 4
The patient shown above is a 72-year-old who has recently undergone neurosurgery.

What abnormality is shown?

Answer 3

A Acne rosacea

B Complications include:
blepharitis,
keratitis,
rhinophyma.

This condition is the result of over-activity of the sebaceous glands, but unlike acne vulgaris, there are no comedones present. Affects forehead, nose, cheeks and chin.

Answer 4
Left 'surgical' third nerve palsy only affecting pupil (dilated) and partial ptosis without ophthalmoplegia.

Question 5

This patient presented with a Bell's palsy.

A What is the name of the unifying syndrome?

B What is the underlying cause?

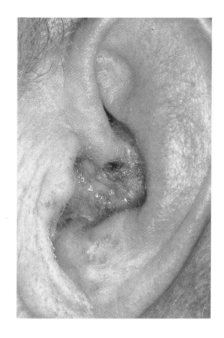

Question 6

This 33-year-old female has a positive VDRL test.

A What is the investigation shown?

B What abnormality is shown?

C What is the likely underlying cause?

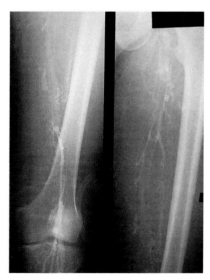

Answer 5

A Ramsay–Hunt syndrome

B Herpes zoster

The Ramsay–Hunt syndrome results from herpetic involvement of the geniculate ganglion of the seventh cranial nerve, resulting in herpetic vesicles at the auditory meatus, tympanic membrane and fauces. Deafness, vertigo and tinnitus may also occur.

Answer 6

A Venogram.

B Femoral deep vein thrombosis.

C Anti-phospholipid syndrome with false positive syphilis serology and thrombotic tendency.

Question 7

This patient presented with nocturia, polyuria and polydipsia. On examination, he is found to be hypertensive and has a bitemporal hemianopia.

A What abnormalities are shown in the radiograph?

B What is the likely underlying diagnosis?

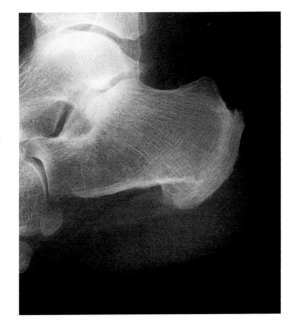

Question 8

This 32-year-old patient presented with a painful proximal myopathy.

What is the diagnosis?

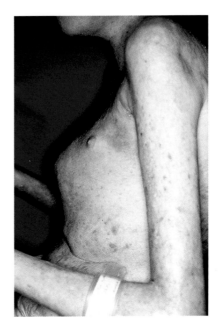

Answer 7

A Calcified plantar fascia; increased heel pad thickness (>22 mm in females; >25 mm in males).

B This patient presented with a history consistent with diabetes mellitus; given the radiographic abnormalities, the likely underlying cause is acromegaly.

Answer 8
Dermatomyositis.

The 'sunburn' rash seen on the exposed part of the chest and the upper arms is typical of the photosensitive rash of dermatomyositis.

Question 9

A   Describe what you see.

B   Give four causes of this abnormality.

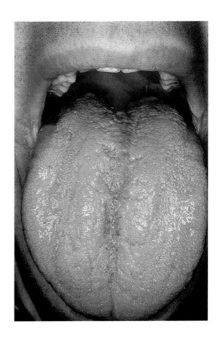

Question 10
What is the likely cause of this
abnormality?

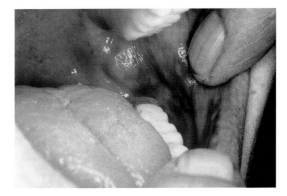

Answer 9

A Macroglossia.

B Causes include:
amyloidosis,
acromegaly,
hypothyroidism,
Down's syndrome,
Duchenne muscular dystrophy.

Answer 10
The slide demonstrates buccal pigmentation due to underlying Addison's disease.

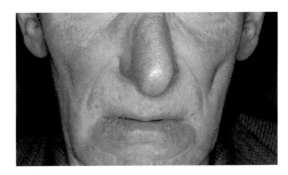

Question 11

This 56-year-old male presented with hypothyroidism FT$_4$ 8 pmol/L, FT$_3$ 1 pmol/L, TSH 20 mU/L.

What is the cause of his abnormal appearance?
(Normal range FT$_3$ 2.8–7.1 pmol/L
              FT$_4$ 13–30 pmol/L
              TSH 0.3–6.0 mU/L)

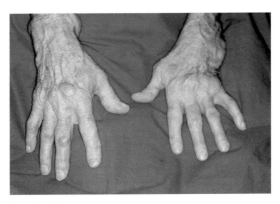

Question 12

Give five abnormal features of the hands shown here.

Answer 11

The subject has the classical slate-grey appearance associated with amiodarone treatment. This drug has several other side-effects, including corneal microdeposits, photosensitivity and pulmonary fibrosis. Abnormal thyroid function tests may also occur. Amiodarone initially blocks the conversion of T_4 to T_3. In the medium term, hypothyroidism may occur. In the longer term, or in patients with a nodular goitre, hyperthyroidism may occur.

Answer 12

The hand shows typical rheumatoid changes, which include:
enlargement of MCP joints,
ulnar deviation,
wasting of the small muscles of the hand bilaterally,
rheumatoid nodules,
Boutonnière deformity of the fifth finger bilaterally.

Question 13

This 35-year-old male presented with recurrent nose bleeds.

A What is this investigation?

B What is the likeliest diagnosis?

C What is the mode of inheritance of this condition?

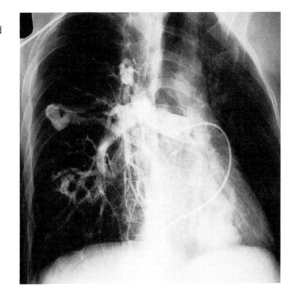

Question 14

Give five complications of the condition shown here.

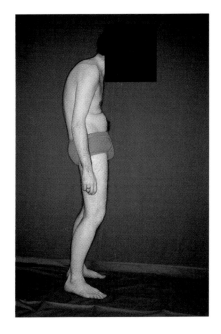

Answer 13

A Pulmonary angiogram.

B Osler–Weber–Rendu syndrome (hereditary haemorrhagic telangiectasia).

C Autosomal dominant.

The pulmonary angiogram shows multiple arterio-venous malformations, which, together with the history of recurrent nose bleeds, is highly suggestive of Osler–Weber–Rendu syndrome in this age group. Pulmonary AV malformations occur in up to 15% of individuals with this syndrome.

Answer 14

Typical features of ankylosing spondylitis are shown, including increased kyphosis, loss of lumbar lordosis and a 'question mark' facies.

Complications of this condition include:
enthesopathy, manifesting as plantar fasciitis and Achille's tendinitis,
aortic incompetence,
apical lung fibrosis leading to a restrictive lung picture,
anterior uveitis,
amyloidosis,
chronic prostatitis,
Cauda Equina syndrome.

Question 15

This 36-year-old asthmatic male presented with collapse and shortness of breath. He was found to be hypotensive.

A What abnormalities are seen in this chest radiograph?

B What is the likely underlying diagnosis?

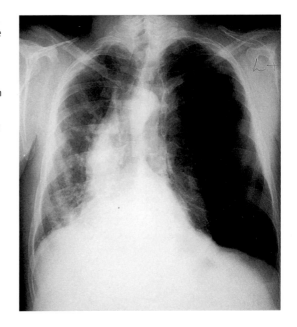

Question 16

A What is the cause of the appearance shown here?

B Give five possible underlying causes.

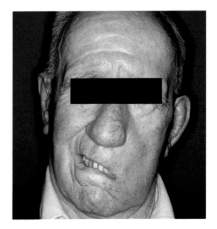

Answer 15

A Significant mediastinal and diaphragmatic displacement to the right due to left-sided pneumothorax.

B Left tension pneumothorax.

Answer 16

A Left lower motor neurone VII nerve palsy.

B Bell's palsy.
Cerebello-pontine angle lesion, e.g. acoustic neuroma.
Diseases affecting seventh nerve as it traverses the parotid gland, e.g. lymphoma, salivary neoplasm, sarcoidosis.
Trauma.
Mononeuritis multiplex.

Question 17

This double contrast study was carried out in a 65-year-old male.

What abnormality is shown?

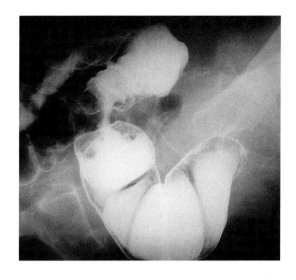

Question 18

A percutaneous cholangiogram was performed on a 38-year-old female who presented with jaundice.

What abnormality is shown?

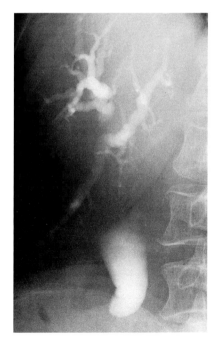

Answer 17

A shouldered lesion with mucosal destruction, giving an 'apple core' appearance, is seen. This would be consistent with a colonic carcinoma.

Answer 18

Obstructed and dilated common bile duct and intrahepatic ducts.

Question 19

A Describe what you see.

B What is the most likely cause.

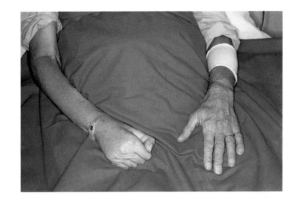

Question 20

This 85-year-old man presented with pyrexia, haemoptysis, weight loss and cough.

A What are the significant radiological findings?

B What is the differential diagnosis?

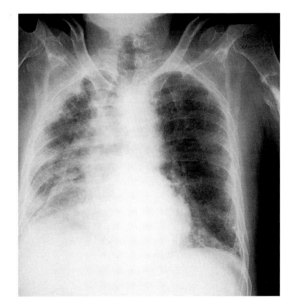

Answer 19

A Generalized wasting of the forearm and intrinsic muscles of the hand. Flexion at the elbow and unopposed flexion of MCP and DIP joints, is also seen.

B Long standing changes from a right sided hemiplegia.

Answer 20

A Right apical fibrosis; volume loss; pleural thickening.

B Re-activation of old tuberculosis/ bronchogenic carcinoma causing partial right upper lobe collapse.

Question 21

This 68-year-old presented with increasing shortness of breath and weight loss.

What procedure has been carried out?

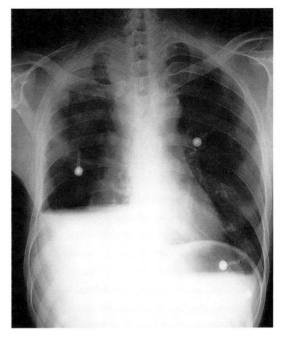

Question 22

This 68-year-old female suffering from rheumatoid arthritis had her drug therapy changed recently.

A What condition is she suffering from?

B What drug did she recently start?

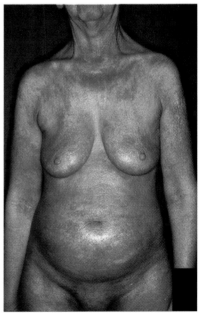

Answer 21
Pleural tap resulting in a right hydropneumothorax.

Answer 22

A Erythroderma or exfoliative dermatitis.

B Gold

Erythroderma can complicate other skin conditions, such as dermatitis and psoriasis; can occur secondary to lymphoma or be a reaction to drugs, e.g. sulphonamides or gold. It is an exfoliative dermatitis that can involve the entire skin surface, causing it to be oedematous and scaly in appearance.

Question 23

The patient shown here presented with a one-week history of fever and cough productive of green sputum.

What is the likely underlying condition and which segment of the lung is affected?

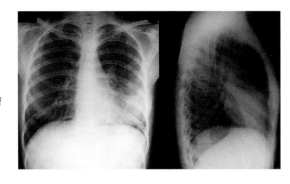

Question 24

What operative procedure has been performed in this 54-year-old female?

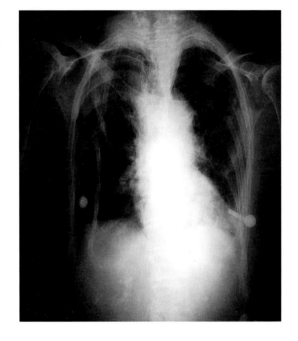

Answer 23

The short history and green sputum is suggestive of a bacterial pneumonia, in this case affecting the superior and inferior segments of the lingula.

Answer 24

Right radical mastectomy with partial rib cage resection.

Question 25

This 76-year-old female presented with shortness of breath on exertion and orthopnoea.

A What abnormality is shown on the chest radiograph?

B What is the likely aetiology of her heart failure?

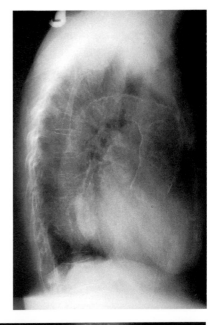

Question 26

What procedure has been carried out on this patient?

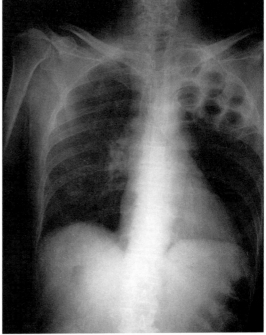

Answer 25

A Calcified, aneurysmal ascending aorta and aortic arch, with cardiomegaly.

B Co-existing aortic regurgitation.

This woman had severe luetic (syphilitic) aortitis, with a thoracic aortic aneurysm, resulting in incompetence of the aortic valve.

Answer 26
Plombage.

This treatment, in addition to thoracoplasty, was fashionable in the early 20th century for tuberculosis.

Question 27
This 65-year-old male presented with left-sided ptosis and miosis.

A What pertinent abnormalities are shown on the radiograph?

B What syndrome does he manifest?

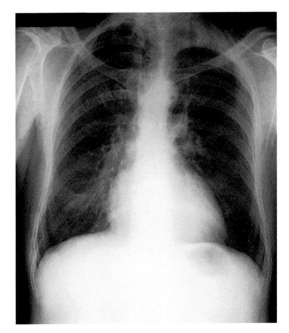

Answer 27

A Left upper lobe mass: probable bronchogenic carcinoma; rib erosion at left upper lobe

B Horner's syndrome

Horner's syndrome results from interruption of the sympathetic nerve supply to the eye, causing partial ptosis (full ptosis is secondary to involvement of the third nerve) and miosis. The sympathetic fibres can be affected at several points on exiting the spinal cord, giving a variety of causes of Horner's syndrome. The example shown here is due to a probable left upper lobe bronchogenic, or Pancoast, tumour.

Question 28

The patient shown here presented with recurrent chest pain at rest.

What is the likely underlying aetiology?

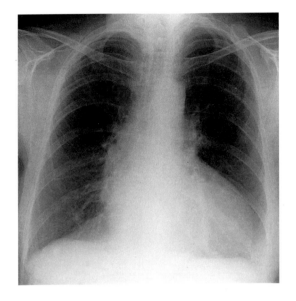

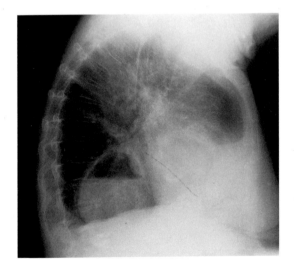

Answer 28
Hiatus hernia

The postero-anterior chest radiograph shows a widened mediastinum with a double right heart border. The wall of the oesophagus is visible through the mediastinal shadow and the stomach bubble is absent, making hiatus hernia the likeliest cause (although achalasia should be considered). The lateral chest radiograph shows the fundus of the stomach as an air–fluid interface behind the heart.

Question 29

This patient presented with fever and bloody diarrhoea.

What is the likely underlying cause of the abnormality shown?

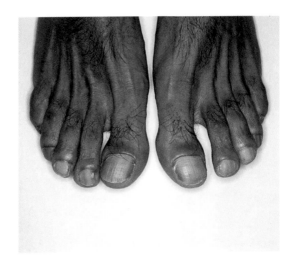

Question 30

This 68-year-old smoker presented with haemoptysis and weight loss.

What abnormality is shown?

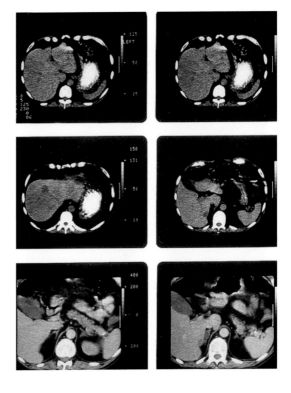

Answer 29
The slide shows clubbing of the toes. Given the history, inflammatory bowel disease is the likely cause of clubbing in this case.

Answer 30
This CT scan of the liver shows multiple lesions in the liver, which, from the history, are probably metastases of a bronchogenic origin.

Question 31

This 68-year-old patient developed a lesion after an ear infection in her teens. She is looking at a red pin on her left.

What is the name given to the syndrome she exemplifies?

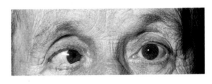

Question 32

Give three possible causes for the chest radiographic abnormality shown here.

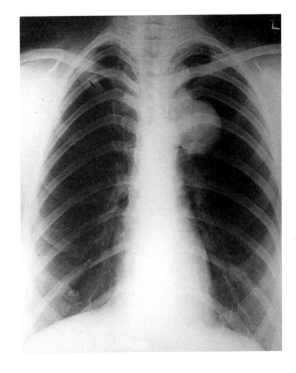

Answer 31

Gradenigo's syndrome.

The patient has a left-sided sixth nerve palsy, with absence of lateral gaze on the affected side. Gradenigo's syndrome is the term used to describe a sixth nerve palsy, caused by involvement of the sixth nerve as it crosses the tip of the petrous temporal bone, subsequent to a middle ear infection.

Answer 32

A 'coin lesion' is seen at the left hilum. This is most likely to be a bronchogenic cyst. Other possibilities for a solitary lung nodule of this size include:
bronchial carcinoma or metastases,
benign bronchial neoplasm, e.g. adenoma, harmatoma,
encysted interlobular effusion,
AV malformation,
pulmonary infarction,
hydatid cyst,
pneumonia,
aspergilloma,
granuloma.

Question 33
What abnormality is shown here?

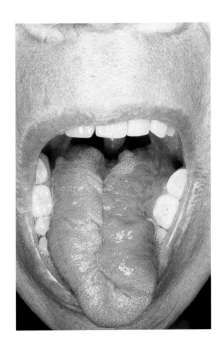

Question 34

A 36-year-old homosexual male presented in casualty with fever and confusion. A lumbar puncture is performed and the organism shown here is isolated (India ink stain).

A What is the organism?

B What treatment would you consider?

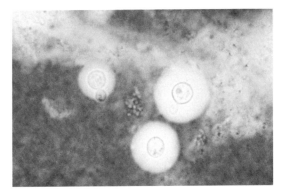

Answer 33

Left twelfth nerve palsy with atrophy of the left side of the tongue and deviation to the affected side.

Answer 34

A *Cryptococcus neoformans*.

B Intravenous amphotericin or fluconazole.

Question 35

What would be your immediate management for this patient?

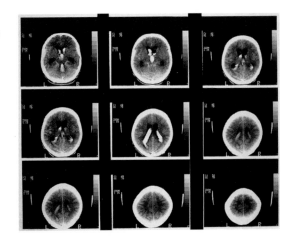

Question 36

This 46-year-old presented with haematuria, weight loss and fever.

What is the likely underlying diagnosis?

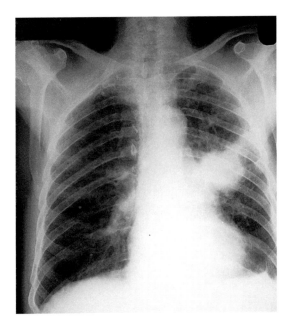

Answer 35
This slide shows a massive subarachnoid haemorrhage. The current management for this is:
intravenous or oral nimodipine (60 mg, four hourly),
bed rest and analgesia,
intravenous rehydration (2–3 l/day) with normal saline, in order to maintain CVP > 10 cm water,
early referral to neurosurgical centre for angiography and consideration of aneurysm clipping.

Answer 36
Cannon ball metastasis from underlying renal cell carcinoma.

Question 37
This 32-year-old was seen in clinic with hypertension.

What is the likely cause?

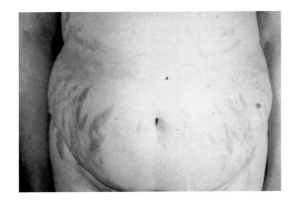

Question 38
A 35-year-old man presented with a swollen left arm three months after a short stay in the intensive care unit.

A What investigation is shown?

B What is the abnormality?

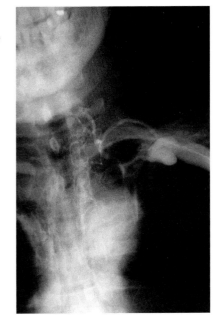

Answer 37

The striae seen in this slide are very suggestive of pituitary Cushing's disease as a cause of this patient's hypertension. They are pigmented, which commonly occurs due to the pituitary secretion of ACTH with MSH. In patients taking oral steroids, pigmentation is less likely as ACTH secretion is suppressed.

Answer 38

A Venogram.

B Left subclavian vein thrombosis (probably as a result of multiple intracaval line insertion) with formation of a collateral circulation.

Question 39
What is the likely diagnosis?

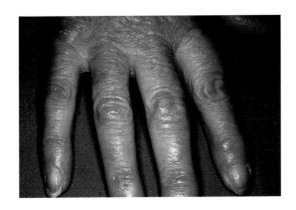

Question 40

A What condition is shown here?

B What is its endocrine association?

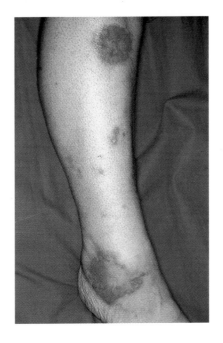

Answer 39

Dermatomyositis.

The hand in the picture shows Gottron's papules over the knuckles with streaking of the extensor tendons. Other changes seen in dermatomyositis include nail fold capillary dilatation, cutaneous calcification and a heliotrope rash over the eyelids and cheeks.

Answer 40

A Necrobiosis lipoidica diabeticorum.

B Diabetes mellitus.

Necrobiosis lipoidica diabeticorum is a painless, yellow-pigmented lesion surrounded by atrophic skin and telangiectasiae. It may be idiopathic in origin but may also be associated with diabetes mellitus and may precede other clinical manifestations of this disorder.

Question 41

This 40-year-old man was referred to an outpatient clinic with hypertension.

A Describe two abnormalities in the skull radiograph shown.

B What is the likely underlying cause of these abnormalities?

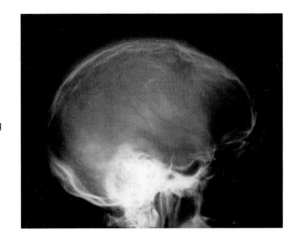

Question 42

Suggest two possible causes of this appearance.

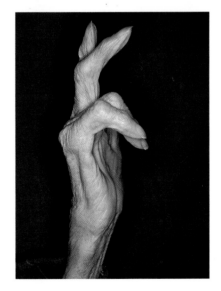

Answer 41

A Enlarged frontal sinuses; double-floored pituitary fossa.

B Acromegaly.

Plain skull radiographs of acromegaly show an enlarged sella turcica in up to 90% of individuals. The double floor effect is due to uneven downward extension of the acidophil adenoma. Other features include destruction of the anterior and posterior clinoids, thickening of the calvarium, enlargement of the paranasal sinuses and prognathism with widening of the mandibular angle. Hypertension, as in this individual, occurs in about a third of cases and is associated with an expanded blood volume and total body sodium.

Answer 42
Dupuytren's contracture/ Ulnar Claw Hand.

Question 43
This 38-year-old female presented with
hypercalcaemia.

A What is the rash shown?

B What is the likely underlying condition?

C Give three other causes of such an appearance.

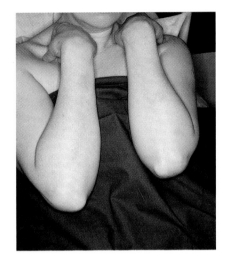

Question 44
This 15-year-old boy presented with a mild fever,
postauricular and cervical lymphadenopathy,
and petechial lesions on the soft palate. The rash
shown here was also present on his forehead and
trunk.

A What is the likely diagnosis?

B What eponymous name is given to the soft
palate lesions?

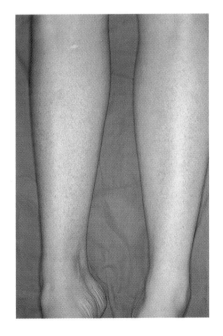

Answer 43

A Erythema nodosum.

B Sarcoidosis.

C Other causes of erythema nodosum include:
infections, e.g. tuberculosis, leprosy, atypical pneumonia,
drugs, e.g. oral contraceptive pill,
inflammatory bowel disorder.

Answer 44

A Rubella.

B Forcheimer spots.

Before immunization was introduced, rubella had a peak incidence amongst teenagers and occurred in both sexes. In the UK, females are now immunized from the age of 11 years. MMR vaccine was introduced for all babies at the age of 13 months. By the year 2003, it is projected that all females in the UK will be immune. Active rubella in pregnant females causes congenital malformations.

The typical signs of rubella infection include conjunctivitis and lymphadenopathy in cervical and posterior auricular sites. Forcheimer spots of the soft palate are suggestive and not diagnostic. The rash itself is pink, discrete and macular, over the forehead, arms and trunk. Splenomegaly may occur.

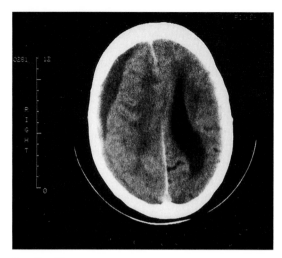

Question 45
The above scan was taken of a 62-year-old male vagrant.

A What is the cause of this man's collapse?

B What drug therapy may improve his consciousness level?

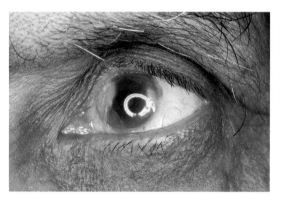

Question 46
The man shown above was a recent immigrant to UK from Sudan.

What abnormality is shown?

Answer 45

A Right-sided subdural haematoma.

B Dexamethasone and mannitol.

The scan shows a subdural haemorrhage with mass effect.

Answer 46
Pterygium.

This is the name applied to a fleshy conjunctival overgrowth over the nasal part of the cornea. It has an association with hot, dry and dusty environments.

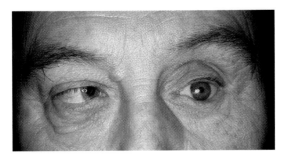

Question 47

This patient is looking to the left. Give the likely cause of the ocular abnormality demonstrated.

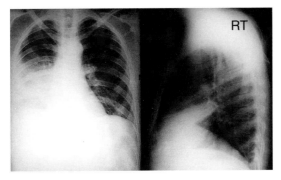

Question 48

This 48-year-old presented with pneumonia.

Which lobe of the lung is affected?

Answer 47

Glass eye on the left-hand side. Note the lack of blood vessels crossing the sclera and the relatively meiotic pupil as compared to the right eye.

Answer 48

Right middle lobe consolidation with loss of right heart border.

Question 49

This man was complaining of long-standing pain in his hands and feet. What is the underlying diagnosis?

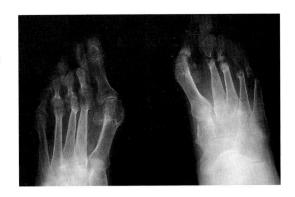

Question 50

This patient was being treated for meningitis.

A What is the rash shown?

B What is the likely precipitant in this case?

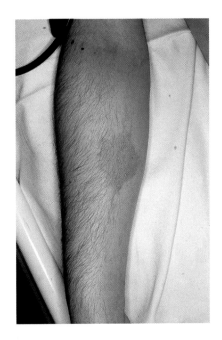

Answer 49

Rheumatoid arthritis.

The radiograph shown illustrates gross rheumatoid changes in the foot. These include osteopenia, loss of joint space, cyst formation in the bone (left second and third metatarsals), 'mouse bite' bone erosions (best seen in the head of the first metatarsal), and destruction of the bone ends with joint ankylosis.

Answer 50

A Fixed drug eruption.

B Penicillin.

Other causes of fixed drug eruptions include sulphonamides and phenolphthalein.

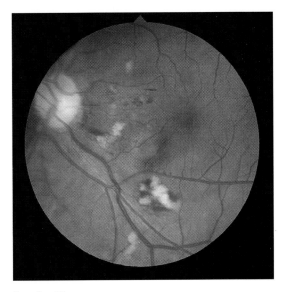

Question 51

A Give three abnormal features seen in the fundal photograph shown above.

B What is the diagnosis?

C What treatment is required?

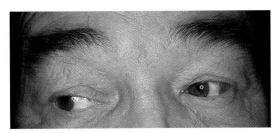

Question 52
What abnormality is shown in this hypertensive male?

Answer 51

A Hard exudates
   Cotton wool spots.
   Microaneurysms.
   Blot haemorrhages.

B The appearances are those of pre-proliferative diabetic retinopathy.

C Pan-retinal photocoagulation is indicated.

Answer 52
Subconjunctival haemorrhage.

This results from rupture of the conjunctival veins allowing extravasation of blood into the potential space between the conjunctiva and Tenon's capsule. Causes include trauma, strangulation and extreme Valsalva manoeuvres, blood dyscrasias and hypertension.

Question 53

The patient shown here is a 35-year-old diabetic.

A What abnormality is shown?

B Give four other conditions, which may cause this abnormality.

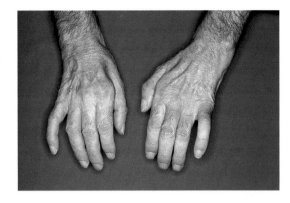

Question 54

The 62-year-old shown here presented with weight loss and a chronic cough.

Give three abnormalities in the chest radiograph shown here and the likely underlying diagnosis.

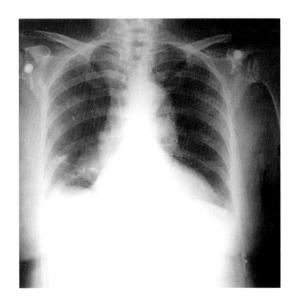

Answer 53

A Bilateral ulnar nerve lesions. There is hyperextension of both fifth metocarpophalyngeal joints with clawing of the hands. There is also wasting of the first dorsal interosseus and some guttering of the remaining interossei.

B Other causes of mononeuritis multiplex include:
leprosy,
connective tissue diseases, e.g. systemic lupus erythematosus (SLE),
sarcoidosis,
malignancy,
amyloidosis,
AIDS,
neurofibromatosis.

Answer 54
Widened mediastinum.
Right middle lobe mass.
Calcified aorta.

In view of the history and age of the patient, the mass is likely to be an underlying bronchial carcinoma.

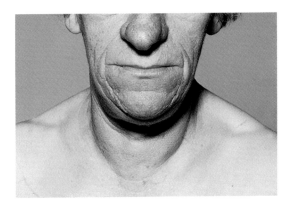

Question 55

A What visual field abnormality might you expect to find in this female?

B What clinical features would allow you to determine whether the patient's disease is active?

C What investigations would assist in confirming the diagnosis?

D What treatment options are available?

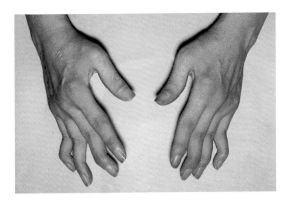

Question 56
What deformity is shown?

Answer 55

A Bitemporal hemianopia.

This patient has a typical acromegalic facies. The underlying acidophil adenoma may cause chiasmatic compression affecting the optic nerve fibres emanating from the nasal retinal fields.

B Glycosuria, sweaty palms and hypertension.

C Glucose tolerance test and CT scan of the pituitary fossa.

D Transphenoidal hypophysectomy, radiotherapy, bromocriptine or octreotide.

Answer 56
Bilateral swan-neck deformities resulting from rheumatoid arthritis.

Question 57

This 58-year-old male presented with a left-sided Horner's syndrome.

A What physical signs are demonstrated?

B What is the likely underlying cause of his problems?

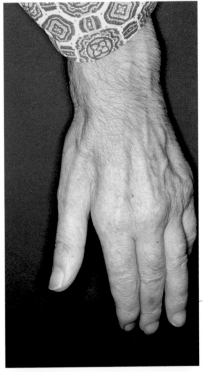

Question 58

This 32-year-old female went on to develop target lesions over her arms a week later.

A What pathology is shown?

B What condition did she develop?

C Give one ocular complication.

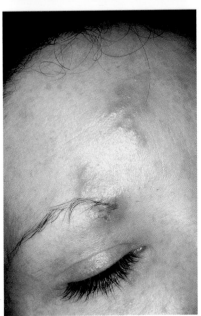

Answer 57

A Nicotine-staining and wasting of the intrinsic hand muscles.

B The photograph shows wasting of the small muscles of the hand with a nicotine-stained middle finger. Together with the history of Horner's syndrome, this constellation of signs is very likely due to a Pancoast's tumour at the left apex causing wasting of T1 muscles, loss of sensation in the T1 dermatome and a left-sided Horner's lesion.

Answer 58

A Herpes simplex lesions over forehead and eyebrow.

B Erythema multiforme.

C Keratitis.

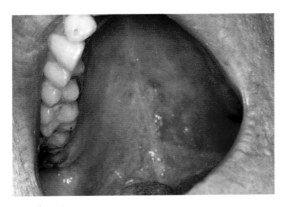

Question 59

What condition is shown?

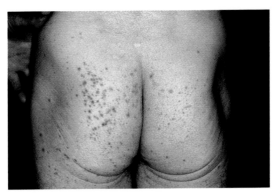

Question 60

This 15-year-old girl presented with abdominal pain and arthritis.

A What condition is shown?

B What alteration of the serum complement level would you expect in this condition?

Answer 59

Herpes zoster: the vesicles shown have a strict dermatomal distribution over one half of the fauces only.

Answer 60

A Henoch–Schonlein purpura.

B Normal serum complement levels.

This condition affects mainly children, often following an upper respiratory tract infection. The features are a purpuric rash, arthritis, abdominal pain, and haematuria. The arthritis, which is flitting in nature, affects mainly the knees and ankles. Renal involvement occurs with nephritic or a nephrotic state. Glomerulonephritis may complicate 30% of cases with 1% of cases proceeding to renal failure.

Question 61

What abnormality is shown in the aortogram?

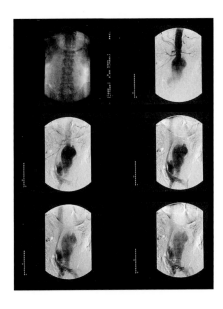

Question 62

This 65-year-old male presented with hypertension and an ulnar nerve lesion on the right-hand side.

What is the likely underlying diagnosis?

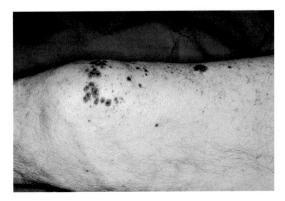

Answer 61

Aortic aneurysm with drainage into the inferior vena cava via a fistula. The renal arteries can be seen above the aneurysm in film number 2 of the sequence.

Answer 62

Polyarteritis nodosa.

This rare condition most often affects middle-aged men. Pathologically, there is microaneurysm formation and fibrinoid necrosis of affected blood vessels. It can present with fever, weight loss, myalgia, arthralgia and a typical vasculitic rash, as shown in this slide. Complications include hypertension, mononeuritis multiplex and renal impairment.

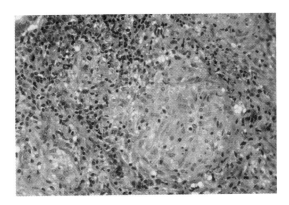

Question 63

This lymph node biopsy is from a 45-year-old man.

A What abnormality is shown?

B Give five causes of this abnormal pathology.

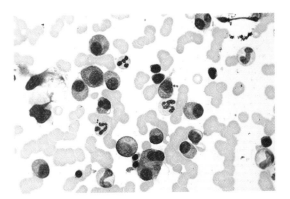

Question 64

The bone marrow aspirate shown above was taken from a 70-year-old man presenting with nausea and abdominal pain.

What is the underlying abnormality?

Answer 63

A Granulomata

B Sarcoidosis.
Tuberculosis.
Hodgkin's lymphoma.
Primary biliary cirrhosis.
Brucellosis.
Histoplasmosis.
Drugs, e.g. sulphonamides.
Berylliosis.

Answer 64

This bone marrow shows a plasma cell infiltrate. These are recognizable by their basophilic cytoplasm and eccentric nuclei with a perinuclear halo. Multiple myeloma causes hypercalcaemia, which caused the abdominal pain in this instance.

Question 65

This 45-year-old female presented with weight loss and a rash.

A Give the name of this condition.

B Give three possible underlying causes.

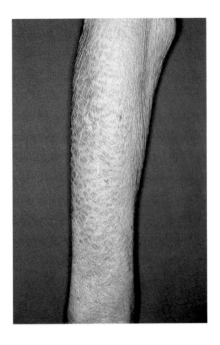

Question 66

What is this condition?

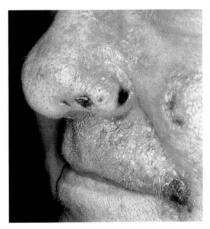

Answer 65

A Acquired ichthyosis

B Hodgkin's disease.
Other malignancies, e.g. Kaposi's sarcoma.
Malnutrition.
Leprosy.

Ichthyosis is characterized by dry and scaly skin in a 'crocodile-skin' type pattern. It may be acquired, as above, or congenital, with either an autosomal dominant or a sex-linked recessive inheritance pattern.

Answer 66
Impetigo.

This skin infection is secondary to staphylococcal or streptococcal infection.

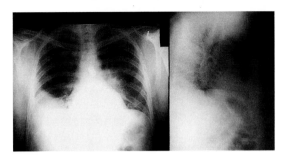

Question 67

This 55-year-old presented with shortness of breath following a cold. He had a decreased percussion note at the right base with a diminution of breath sounds over the same area.

What radiological abnormality is seen at the base of the right lung?

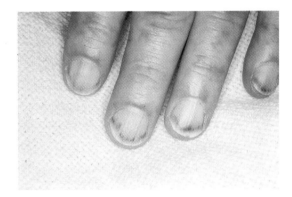

Question 68

This 40-year-old female presented with fever, weight loss and shortness of breath on exertion. On examination, she has an early diastolic murmur audible at the left sternal edge.

A What abnormality is shown?

B What is the likely underlying pathology?

Answer 67

Collapse of the right lower lobe of the lung.

Answer 68

A Splinter haemorrhages.

B Infective endocarditis.

Although infective endocarditis is the most likely diagnosis in this case, other conditions that may result in splinter haemorrhages include SLE. This is also a possibility in this case where pneumonitis may have resulted in respiratory symptoms.

Question 69

This 15-year-old boy has Crohn's disease. What abnormality is shown?

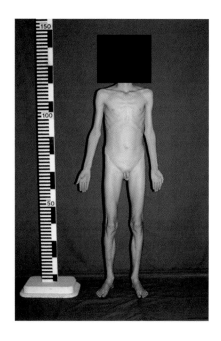

Question 70

This 80-year-old female presented with polyuria and malaise.

A What condition is shown?

B What is the likely underlying diagnosis?

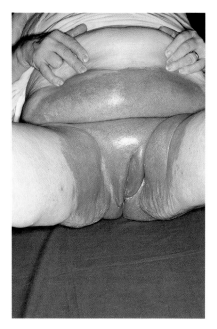

Answer 69

Delayed puberty due to chronic illness (note sparse secondary sexual hair and under-developed genitalia). This boy's bone age was 10.

Answer 70

A Intertrigo.

B Diabetes mellitus.

Intertrigo is a red flexural rash secondary to candidiasis with a fringe of vesicles, pustules and scales. Diabetes is suggestive from the history of polyuria secondary to an osmotic diuresis, and is a risk factor for fungal infections.

Question 71
What renal abnormality does the intravenous
urogram shown here demonstrate?

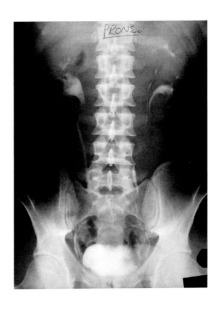

Question 72
What abnormality is shown?

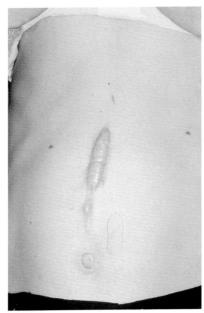

Answer 71

Duplex collecting system on the left-hand side.

Answer 72

Keloid formation at the site of a scar. This is more common in people of Afro-Caribbean origin.

Question 73
This 30-year-old male presented with fever and
weight loss.

What lesion is shown here?

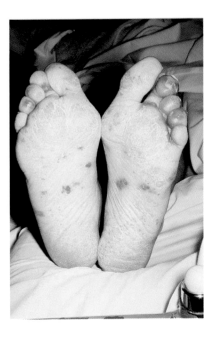

Question 74
What is the differential
diagnosis of the lesion shown
here?

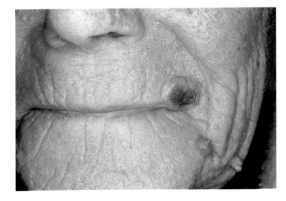

Answer 73
Kaposi's sarcoma on the feet of a patient with AIDS.

Answer 74
Keratoacanthoma.
Squamous cell carcinoma.

Keratoacanthomas are benign tumours thought to arise from hair follicles. They have a central keratinous plug and have a very similar histological appearance to squamous cell carcinomata. Their clinical course is, however, different in that they spontaneously involute leaving a residual scar at the site.

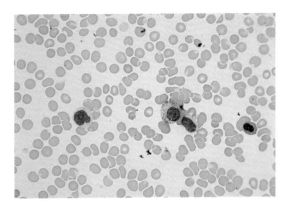

Question 75

The blood film shown here is from a 68-year-old male who presented with haemoptysis and coughing. On abdominal examination there is no organomegaly present.

A What does the blood film show?

B What is the underlying pathology?

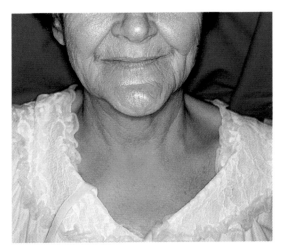

Question 76

This 58-year-old presented with pruritis. Her IgM level was markedly elevated.

What is the likely underlying diagnosis?

Answer 75

A Leukoerythroblastic blood film: nucleated red blood cell and myelocyte forms present.

B Bronchial carcinoma with bony metastases.

A leukoerythroblastic blood film may occur as a result of many diverse conditions. If splenomegaly is clinically apparent, the underlying condition may be myelofibrosis or lymphoma. If splenomegaly is absent, the possibilities include myeloma, acute leukaemia and carcinomatosis. In this example, metastatic invasion of the bone marrow has caused release of cell precursors, such as myelocytes, metamyelocytes and normoblasts, into the general circulation, resulting in a leukoerythroblastic blood film.

Answer 76
Primary biliary cirrhosis.

This patient is frankly icteric. This, coupled with her sex, age group, presentation with pruritis and elevated IgM, suggests that she is very likely to have primary biliary cirrhosis. Other features of this condition include osteoporosis, osteomalacia and hypercholesterolaemia manifested by xanthelasmata. Biochemical tests show an elevated alkaline phosphatase and antimitochondrial antibodies may also be detected.

Question 77

A What type of scan is shown here?

B What abnormalities are visible on this scan?

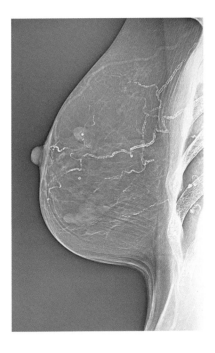

Question 78

The patient shown presented with a meningioma.

A What oral lesion is shown?

B What are the underlying possible conditions with their genomic locations?

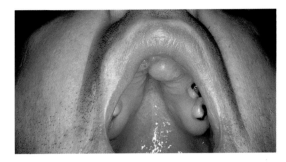

Answer 77

A Xerographic mammogram.

B Two soft lesions are seen. The first is well defined and calcified, and is likely to be a benign fibroadenoma. The other lesion may be another fibroadenoma, but would also be compatible with a lobular carcinoma. There is also calcification of the blood vessels present.

Xerographic mammograms have now been replaced by film screen mammography, which uses lower radiation doses.

Answer 78

A Palatal neurofibromata.

B Neurofibromatosis type I (NF 1), or neurofibromatosis type II (NF 2).
Chromosome 17 and 22 respectively.

There are two types of neurofibromatosis (Von Recklinghausen's syndrome) recognized. Type I, carried on chromosome 17, has peripheral manifestations, presenting with café au lait patches, skin tumours, neural tumours (which include cutaneous neurofibromata) and central nervous system tumours such as meningiomata. Type II, carried on chromosome 22, presents with bilateral acoustic neuromata. Meningiomata may also occur. Oral neurofibromata are seen in 10% of patients with neurofibromatosis.

Question 79

A What abnormality is shown?

B What two simple bedside tests would you conduct?

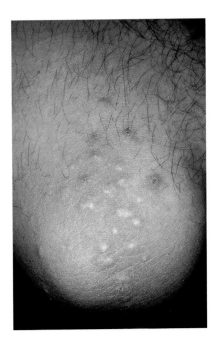

Question 80

A What abnormality is shown here?

B What is the likely underlying process?

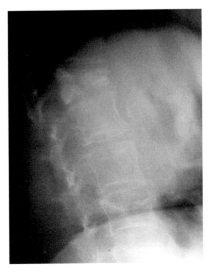

Answer 79

A Eruptive xanthomata around the knee.

B Fundoscopic examination for lipaemia retinalis;
dipstick urine for glucose.

Eruptive xanthomata are multiple red/yellow vesicles that are found on extensor surfaces of the body, e.g. buttocks, elbows, knees and the back. They occur in type IV hyperlipidaemia (familial hypertriglyceridaemia). This is associated with diabetes and obesity. They are also found in type I (lipoprotein lipase deficiency) and in type V (Apo-C II deficiency) hyperlipidaemias.

Answer 80

A Wedge fracture of spinal vertebra.

B Osteoporosis.

Question 81

A What two abnormalities are shown?

B What is the likely underlying diagnosis?

C Give four complications of this condition.

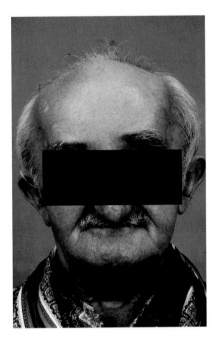

Question 82

The patient shown has nephrotic syndrome.

A What abnormality is shown?

B What is the underlying renal pathology?

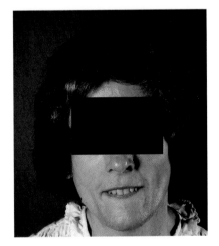

Answer 81

A Hearing aid right ear.
   Prominent forehead.

B Paget's disease.

C Deafness.
   Increased skull thickening.
   Fractures and bone pain.
   Osteogenic sarcoma.
   Cranial nerve compression leading to palsy.

Paget's disease is caused by increased bone turnover, with excessive osteoclastic resorption followed by increased osteoblastic activity. It affects as many as 10% of the population at the age of 70 and has a male-to-female ratio of 2:1. Deafness can be nerve deafness (due to compression of the VIIIth cranial nerve) or conductive deafness, due to Paget's disease involving the ossicles.

Answer 82

A Marked loss of subcutaneous tissue from the face suggestive of partial lipodystrophy.

B Mesangiocapillary glomerulonephritis type II.

Type II mesangiocapillary glomerulonephritis, or dense deposit disease due to the deposition of electron-dense intramembranous material, is characterized by the presence of C3 nephritic factor. The latter stabilizes C3bBb, leading to a reduced C3 and reduced factor B level, with a normal level of C4.

Question 83

A Describe two nail form abnormalities in the slide shown.

B What is the underlying diagnosis?

C Comment on the complexion of the skin.

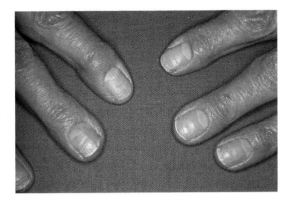

Question 84

This 35-year-old female presented with menorrhagia and the above rash. Physical examination was otherwise unremarkable.

A Suggest a diagnosis.

B What would the bone marrow be expected to show?

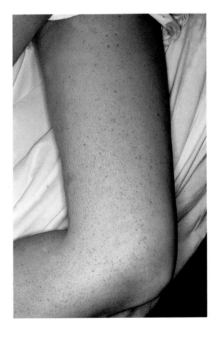

Answer 83

A Onycholysis.
Transverse ridging.

B Psoriasis.

C The patient is tanned after PUVA therapy for his psoriasis.

Answer 84

A Immune thrombocytopenic purpura (ITP).

B Increased megakaryocytes in the bone marrow.

ITP can be acute or chronic in nature. The acute form is seen in young children, usually after a viral infection. The chronic form is usually seen in adult females and is an autoimmune process, with platelet antibodies being identified in 60–70% of affected individuals. Signs include easy bruising, purpura, epistaxis and menorrhagia.

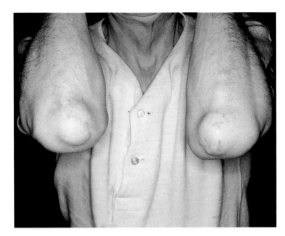

Question 85

What is the differential diagnosis of the lesions shown?

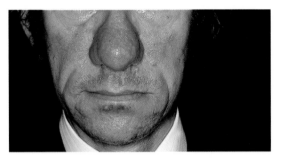

Question 86

The patient shown here presented with shortness of breath.

A What is the differential diagnosis of his skin lesion?

B What is the likeliest cause of his shortness of breath?

Answer 85
Rheumatoid nodules.
Gout.
Tendon xanthomata.

Answer 86

A Lupus pernio associated with pulmonary sarcoidosis/ lupus vulgaris associated with pulmonary tuberculosis.

B Pulmonary fibrosis.

Lupus pernio is a cutaneous manifestation of chronic sarcoidosis, which is often associated with pulmonary fibrosis and uveitis. Lupus vulgaris has an 'apple jelly' appearance when pressed under a microscope slide.

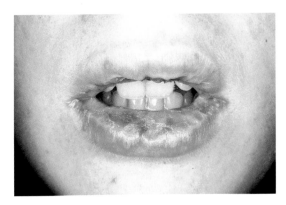

Question 87

The appearance shown above was accompanied by a skin rash.

A What is the name of this syndrome?

B Give four causes of the syndrome.

C What name is given to the skin rash?

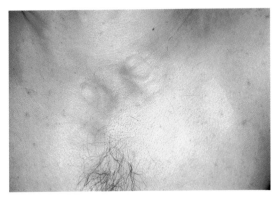

Question 88

This 48-year-old male presented with weight loss and haemoptysis. He had noticed his collar had become increasingly tight a week prior to being seen.

A What abnormality is shown?

B What is the likely cause?

Answer 87

A Stevens–Johnson syndrome.

B Infections: Herpes, *Mycoplasma*, *Streptococcus*.

Drugs: sulphonamides, penicillin, barbiturates, salicylates.

C Erythema multiforme.

Stevens–Johnson syndrome is the combination of erythema multiforme, a systemic illness (manifesting as fever and arthralgia) and ulceration of at least two mucosal surfaces.

Answer 88

A Pitting oedema of the neck.

B Superior vena caval (SVC) obstruction secondary to bronchial carcinoma.

SVC obstruction can present with fullness in the head, facial oedema, shortness of breath and blackouts.

Question 89

This 50-year-old presented with a photosensitive rash, Raynaud's phenomenon and a high ESR. What is the likely diagnosis?

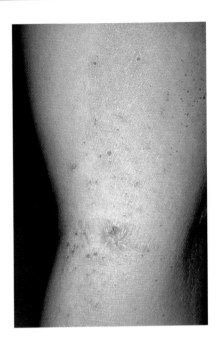

Question 90

What is the cause of the abnormal appearance shown?

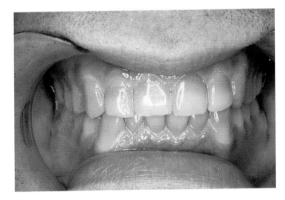

Answer 89

Cutaneous lupus.

This slide shows an erythematous rash with follicular plugging and scarring typical of cutaneous lupus. This condition has a lower female preponderance than SLE and has an older age peak (40–50 years). An arthropathy and Raynaud's phenomenon may occur and full-blown SLE can develop.

Answer 90

Tetracycline exposure causing the staining of teeth and enamel hypoplasia.

Question 91

This 82-year-old male presents with frequent headaches.

A What two abnormalities are apparent?

B What is the likely cause of his headaches?

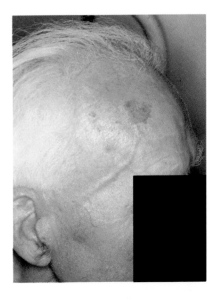

Question 92

This 58-year-old farmer presented with the rash shown here.

A What is the rash shown?

B How may he have acquired it?

C Suggest a treatment for it.

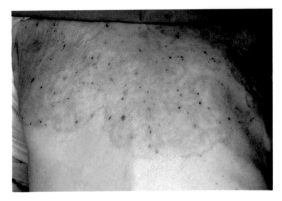

Answer 91

A Visibly thickened temporal artery.
Solar keratosis.

B Temporal arteritis.

Answer 92

A Tinea corporis.

B Contact with cattle infected with *Trichophyton verrucosum*.

C Oral fluconazole.

The rash presented has the typical annular, erythematous lesions—with well-defined edges, studded with papules and pustules—seen with *Tinea* infections of the skin. Farm workers, due to their occupational contact with animals, are particularly at risk of contracting this zoonosis.

Question 93

This 82-year-old male presented with weight loss.
His thyroid function tests were normal.

A What abnormalities are shown here?

B What is the likely cause?

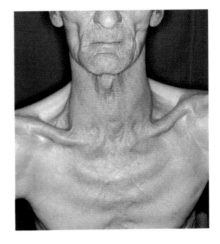

Answer 93

A Goitre.
Emaciation.

B Carcinoma of the thyroid, probably anaplastic.

A nontoxic goitre with weight loss is suggestive of anaplastic carcinoma of the thyroid. This locally invasive tumour has a poor prognosis.

Question 94

This 52-year-old male with pulmonary tuberculosis, having recently finished a course of antituberculous drugs, presented on this occasion with a three-day history of fever, shortness of breath and a cough productive of green sputum.

A What abnormalities are shown on the radiograph?

B What is the likely cause of his acute presentation?

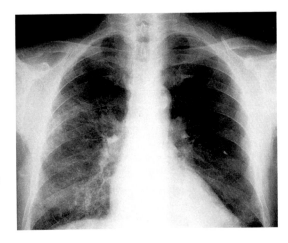

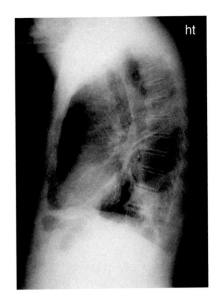

Answer 94

A Right middle and lower lobe interstitial shadowing secondary to tuberculosis.
Left lower lobe collapse and consolidation.

B Pneumococcal pneumonia.

The history and radiographic appearance are suggestive of a bacterial pneumonia. Lobar consolidation is typical of pneumococcal pneumonia; *Klebsiella* can also cause this appearance, but tends to cavitate rapidly and leads to bulging of the fissure. Atypical pneumonias rarely cause lobar consolidation and usually give a bilateral diffuse reticulo-nodular infiltrates.

Left lower lobe collapse is often difficult to see on a PA film but gives the classical 'sail sign' with a straight left heart border. On the lateral film, the greater fissure, usually running from D4/5 and through the hilum to 5 cm behind the sternum, is in this case displaced behind the hilum.

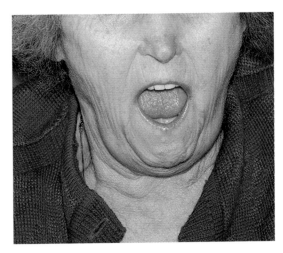

Question 95

What underlying diagnosis is suggested by this facial appearance?

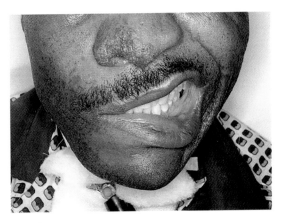

Question 96

This patient presented with the facial appearance, fever and parotid gland enlargement shown here.

What syndrome does he exhibit?

Answer 95

Systemic sclerosis or CREST syndrome.

The female shown has typical facial features for systemic sclerosis or CREST syndrome, with beaking of the nose, absence of facial wrinkles, xerostomia and telangiectasia.

Answer 96

Uveoparotid fever or Heerfordt's syndrome.

This syndrome, due to sarcoidosis, was first described by Heerfordt, a Danish opthalmologist, in 1909, and is the combination of parotid enlargement, fever and uveitis. The patient shown has lupus pernio and a right lower motor neurone VIIth nerve palsy, which can occur with sarcoidosis.

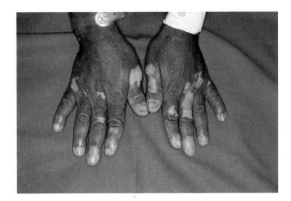

Question 97

A What condition is shown?

B Give three associated disorders.

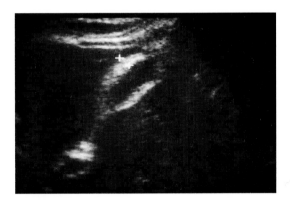

Question 98
This 43-year-old female presented with a three-day history of fever, abdominal pain, vomiting and jaundice.

A What type of scan is shown?

B Name the marked structure.

Answer 97

A Vitiligo.

B Pernicious anaemia.
Grave's disease.
Diabetes mellitus (type I).
Addison's disease.
Primary hypothyroidism.
Achlorhydria.

Vitiligo, i.e. de-pigmentation of the skin, is thought to be an autoimmune-mediated process leading to destruction of the melanocytes, and is associated with a number of other organ-specific, autoimmune disorders. In the active phase of vitiligo, the Koebner phenomenon may occur.

Answer 98

A Ultrasound scan of the abdomen.

B Thickened wall of gall bladder in a case of acute cholangitis. The patient has presented with features of Saint's triad (abdominal pain, fever and jaundice).

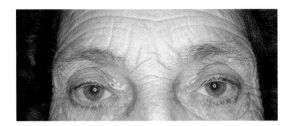

Question 99

The 78-year-old female shown above was treated for hypothermia, having been found unconscious in her flat.

A What abnormality is shown?

B What is the likely underlying disorder?

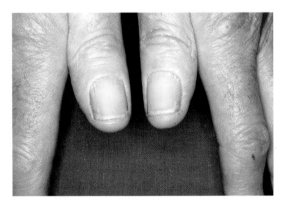

Question 100

A What abnormality is shown?

B Give three associations of this condition.

Answer 99

A Xanthelasmata surrounding the eyes.

B Hypothyroidism.

Hypothyroidism can present acutely in the elderly with hypothermia and coma. Hypothyroidism is associated with hypercholesterolaemia, resulting in the xanthelasmata seen in this case. Other conditions associated with hypercholesterolaemia include diet, cirrhotic liver disease, e.g. primary biliary cirrhosis and nephrotic syndrome.

Answer 100

A Yellow nail syndrome.

B Yellow nail syndrome is characterized by yellow/green nails and is associated with congenital lymphoedema (due to atresia or varicosity of the lymph vessels), pleural effusions, chronic bronchitis, bronchiectasis and chronic sinus infections.

Question 101
This 56-year-old female presented with dysphagia.

A What abnormality is shown?

B What is the likely underlying cause?

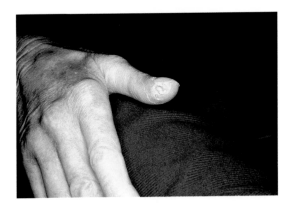

Question 102
This patient complains of nausea, abdominal pain and constipation.

A What corneal abnormality is shown?

B What is the underlying diagnosis?

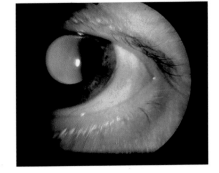

Answer 101

A Calcinosis of the thumb.

B Systemic sclerosis or CREST syndrome.

Systemic sclerosis is a multisystem disorder with a female preponderance, usually presenting in women under the age of 50 years. CREST syndrome, is the combination of calcinosis, Raynaud's disease, oesophageal involvement, sclerodactyly, and telangiectasia. Speckled ANA are found in 60% of systemic sclerosis and the anticentromere antibody is associated with the CREST syndrome. Oesophageal involvement, as in this case, is common, and may be associated with general atony of the small and large bowel.

Answer 102

A Corneal arcus due to calcification.

B Primary hyperparathyroidism leading to hypercalcaemia.

Other causes of hypercalcaemia do not result in arcus or corneal calcification because patients usually do not survive long enough to develop these abnormalities.

Question 103

A What abnormality is shown?

B Give four associated causes.

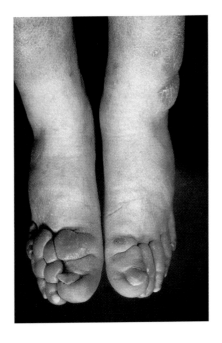

Question 104

The 26-year-old shown here presented with pyrexia and hypotension.

A What abnormality is shown?

B What is the likely underlying cause?

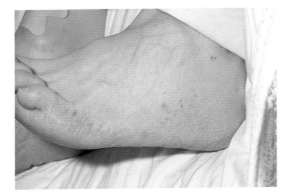

Answer 103

A Lymphoedema of the legs.

Pretibial myxoedema may have a similar appearance but usually involves the medial aspect of the shins.

B Infective, e.g. secondary to *Wuchereia bancroftii*.
Secondary to pelvic trauma, malignancy, radiotherapy.
Congenital.

Answer 104

A Purpuric rash over feet.

B Meningococcal septicaemia.

The case illustrated is a common history for acute menigococcal sepsis, with rapid onset of cardiovascular collapse leading to coma. The purpuric rash is typical; the concomitant gangrene that occurs is often exacerbated by the use of large amounts of noradrenaline as a pressor agent.

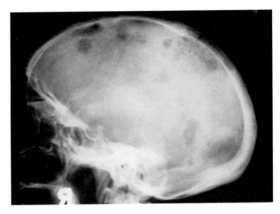

Question 105

A What abnormality is shown?

B What is the underlying disorder?

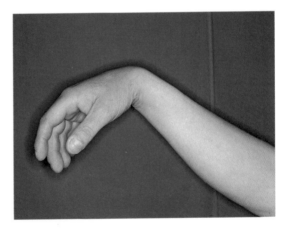

Question 106

The 28-year-old shown above presented after a heavy night's drinking.

A What abnormality is shown, and what is the likely cause?

B What name is commonly given to this condition?

Answer 105

A 'Tam O'Shanter' cap appearance of the skull, with a deformed, thickened vault and osteoporosis circumscripta.

B Underlying Paget's disease of bone.

Paget's disease is thought to be due to excessive osteoclastic resorption of bone, followed by excess osteoblastic activity. The aetiology is unknown. The disease affects 10% of the population above the age of 70 years, and has a male preponderance. The disorder may be entirely asymptomatic, being picked up on routine blood testing, with an otherwise inexplicably raised bone alkaline phosphatase, or may present with painful deformation of the long bones and skull. Osteoporosis circumscripta represents areas of bone porosis and sclerosis.

Answer 106

A Wrist drop secondary to probable radial nerve palsy.

B Saturday night palsy.

Saturday night palsy refers to the scenario of the drunken, stuporous young man spending the night sleeping in a hard chair with his arm draped over the back. This results in compression of the radial nerve against the humeral shaft, causing a radial nerve palsy.

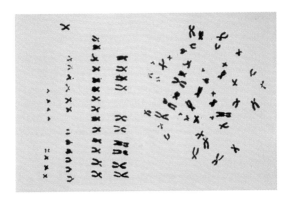

Question 107

A What abnormality is shown?

B What is the likely cause?

C Give three clinical signs that may be apparent.

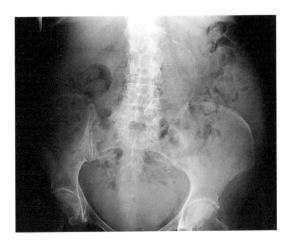

Question 108

A 70-year-old male presented with sudden onset of abdominal pain. On examination he is clinically shocked. What is the diagnosis based on the abdominal radiograph?

Answer 107

A Single X chromosome, with no Y chromosome present.

B Turner's syndrome. Nondysjunction of the X chromosome, resulting in a X45 chromosome number. This gives a negative buccal smear (i.e. no Barr body present) and a typical set of features.

C Typical phenotypic features of this disorder include: short height; cubitus valgus; high-arched palate; short fourth metacarpal; shield chest with widely spaced nipples; lymphoedema; low hairline; poorly developed secondary sexual characteristics, e.g. small breasts and sparse secondary sexual hair. Associated features include primary amenorrhoea, coarctation of the aorta and horse-shoe kidney.

Answers 108

Ruptured abdominal aortic aneurysm.

The abdominal radiograph shows the calcification in the wall of the aneurysm.

Question 109

A What abnormality is shown?

B Give three causative organisms.

C Suggest an appropriate treatment.

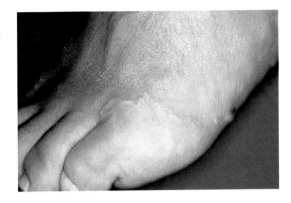

Question 110

This 42-year-old female presented with a dry cough and shortness of breath followed by the rash shown.

A What is the skin lesion shown?

B What is the likely underlying cause?

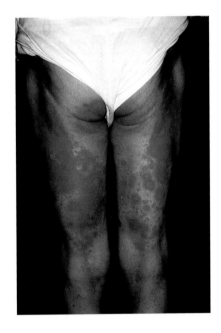

Answer 109

A Cutaneous larva migrans.

B The nematodes responsible for this condition are:
Ankylostoma duodenale and *Necator americanus*—hookworms which are human parasites.
Strongyloides stercoralis—heavy asymptomatic infestations with these worms may occur with
fulminating disease occurring many years later, e.g. former prisoners of war interred in the Far East,
immigrant groups.
Ankylostoma brazilense and *caninum*—cat and dog hookworms which are occasional human
parasites. As they lack the enzymes required to penetrate beyond the skin, their infestations remain
confined to the skin.

C Local or systemic thiabendazole.

Cutaneous larva migrans is a disease of tropical/subtropical climates (this eruption may also be known as
larva currens when seen in strongyloidiasis). The filariform larvae, after emerging from the faeces,
penetrate intact skin, causing intensely itchy blisters ('ground itch') followed two to three days later by the
appearance of a serpiginous creeping eruption, which results from the worms migrating under the skin.
This may be accompanied by urticarial wheals. The disorder is often associated with a systemic
eosinophilia.

Answer 110

A Erythema multiforme.

B *Mycoplasma pneumoniae.*

The typical concentric, erythematous papules of erythema multiforme are shown.

Question 111

This 34-year-old female presented with fever and diarrhoea.

A What two abnormalities are shown?

B What is the likely underlying diagnosis?

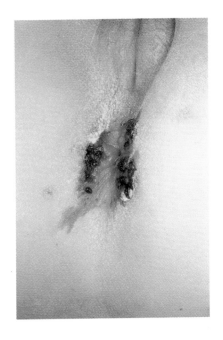

Question 112

This 60-year-old male was on long-term treatment for a cardiac condition.

A What abnormality is shown here?

B What two conditions might he have been treated for?

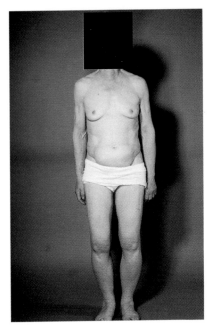

Answer 111

A Perianal tags and fistula formation (the opening of this can be seen to the right of the anus).

B Crohn's disease.

Answer 112

A Gynaecomastia.

B Atrial dysrrhythmia treated with digoxin, or congestive cardiac failure treated with spironolactone.

The causes of gynaecomastia include antiandrogen drugs (e.g. spironolactone and cimetidine), weak oestrogens (e.g. digoxin) and chronic liver disease.

Question 113
What is the underlying condition?

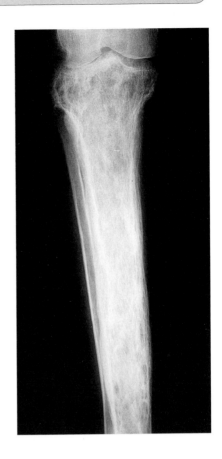

Question 114

A What lesions are shown on the trunk of this 28-year-old male?

B What is the condition in which these lesions may be seen?

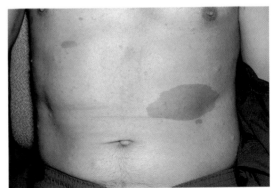

Answer 113

Paget's disease.

The slide shows a Pagetic tibia *en face*. Paget's disease of the long bones causes thickening of the cortices with a combination of lytic areas.

Answer 114

A Café au lait patches and small neurofibromata.

B Neurofibromatosis type 1.

Question 115

The 68-year-old male shown presented with haemoptysis and weight loss.

A What abnormality is shown in his chest radiograph?

B What is the differential diagnosis?

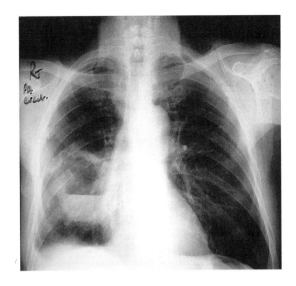

Question 116

The 45-year-old female shown here presented with weight loss and a pyrexia, two weeks after a three-month period travelling through the USA. Her chest radiograph is shown.

What is the differential diagnosis of her underlying condition based on this chest radiograph?

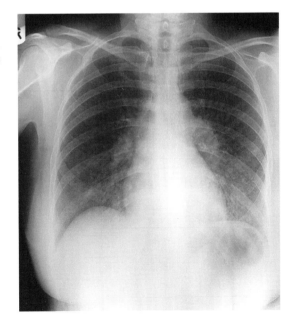

Answer 115

A Cavitating lesion.

B Cavitating squamous carcinoma of the lung.
Infective abscess cavity.

Answer 116
Histoplasmosis.
Blastomycosis.
Cryptococcosis.
Miliary tuberculosis.
Miliary carcinomatosis.

Question 117

This 50-year-old male has a history of ischaemic heart disease.

A What abnormality is shown?

B What is the underlying condition?

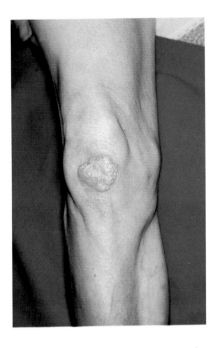

Question 118

This 62-year-old male with known carcinoma of the bronchus, presented with increased shortness of breath on routine follow-up.

A What is the main abnormality shown in the chest radiograph?

B What is the underlying cause?

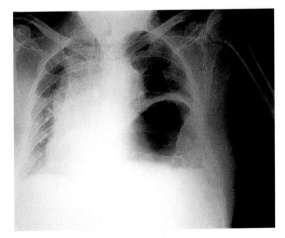

Answer 117

A Tuberose xanthoma over the knee.

B Familial hypercholesterolaemia IIa.

This autosomal dominant condition is due to problems of binding and internalization of the LDL receptor, resulting in elevated serum LDL levels. Homozygotes develop ischaemic heart disease prematurely, in childhood. This subject is a heterozygote.

Answer 118

A Raised left hemidiaphragm.

This CXR is rotated, thereby explaining the apparent mediastinal shift. There is no evidence of lung collapse as the whole lung field can be seen. A concurrent pneumonia cannot, however, be excluded.

B Left phrenic nerve infiltration by bronchial carcinoma.

A raised left hemidiaphragm tends to present with shortness of breath on exertion and flatulence. The commonest cause of a unilateral phrenic nerve paralysis is carcinoma of the bronchus. Bilateral phrenic nerve paralysis may be due to a variety of causes including motor neurone disease, polio, syringomyelia, cervical spondylosis, *herpes zoster*, polyneuropathy and myopathy.

Question 119

The patient shown here had presented the week before to her general practitioner complaining of a runny nose and sore eyes. He had noticed white spots in her mouth on examination.

A What is the underlying condition?

B What eponymous name is given to the white spots?

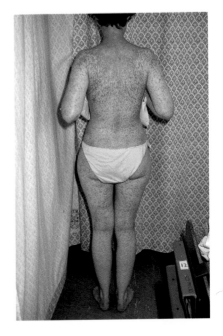

Question 120

A What clinical signs does this patient manifest?

B What is his thyroid status?

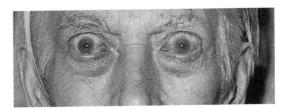

Answer 119

A Measles.

B Koplik's spots.

The differential diagnosis of a viral exanthem is wide and includes infectious mononucleosis, CMV, hepatitis A, B and C, and rubella. However, the coalescing rash and the above history are typical of measles. The prodrome of this illness is a runny nose, sore throat, conjunctivitis and oral Koplik's spots, which are red oral lesions with a central white fleck. The skin manifestations appear one to two weeks later with a morbilliform rash over the head and neck, which then spreads to the trunk and limbs.

Answer 120

A Proptosis.
   Conjunctival oedema.
   Lid retraction.

B The patient may be eu-, hypo- or hyperthyroid.

Opthalmic Grave's disease is due to an antibody causing retro-orbital inflammation and oedema. The oedema may lead to proptosis and this, in turn, may cause conjunctival oedema. Ophthalmic Grave's is often associated with Grave's hyperthyroidism but patients may also be hypo- or euthyroid. Opthalmoplegia may also occur.

Question 121
The 38-year-old male shown presented with
shortness of breath on exertion and fever.

A What condition is shown?

B What is the likely cause of his respiratory
symptoms?

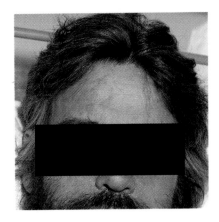

Question 122

A What is the lesion shown?

B What features affect
prognosis?

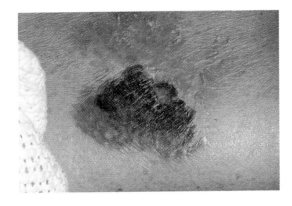

Answer 121

A Seborrhoeic dermatitis.

B *Pneumocystis carinii* pneumonia.

Seborrhoeic dermatitis shown above is associated with HIV disease. PCP pneumonia can be the first manifestation of AIDS, and occurs at least once in 80% of patients with AIDS.

Answer 122

A Superficial spreading malignant melanoma.

B Site: limbs carry a better prognosis than trunk, and trunk better than face.

   Depth of tumour: < 1 mm thick—5 years survival rate > 90%; > 3.5 mm thick—5 years survival rate < 50%.

Question 123

This 60-year-old male suffered from intermittently cold hands, particularly in cold weather.

A What condition is shown?

B What disorders may it be associated with?

C What screening tests would you consider?

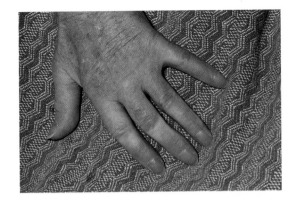

Question 124

This 48-year-old male presented with dysphasia. He was otherwise well.

A What abnormality is shown?

B What other brain locations are commonly affected?

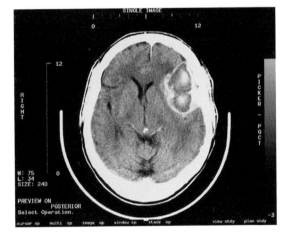

Answer 123

A Raynaud's phenomenon.

B Collagen vascular disease, e.g. scleroderma, rheumatoid arthritis, SLE.
Neurogenic lesions—thoracic outlet syndrome, carpal tunnel syndrome.
Arterial disease—atherosclerosis, thromboangiitis obliterans.
Occupational—vibrating tools.
Miscellaneous—cryoglobulinaemia.

C ANA, ESR, complement titres, serum protein electrophoresis, cryoglobulins, rheumatoid factor, thoracic outlet radiograph, barium swallow.

Answer 124

A Left frontoparietal meningioma.

B Parasagittal, olfactory groove, sphenoid ridge and convexities, and around the sella turcica.

The CT scan shows a high attenuation lesion attached to the meninges, with marked post-contrast enhancement, typical of a meningioma. The lesion is unlikely to have been caused by infections, such as toxoplasmosis, as this man is systemically well.

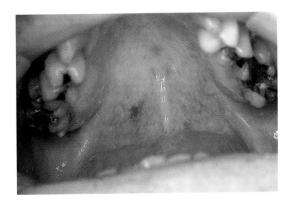

Question 125

This 50-year-old male was suffering from AIDS.

A What abnormality is shown?

B What are the probable causes in this context?

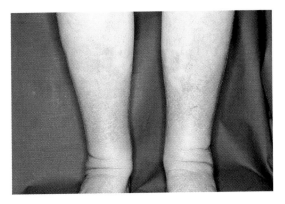

Question 126

This 48-year-old female presented with proptosis of the right eye and weight loss.

A What abnormality is shown?

B What underlying condition does she have?

Answer 125

A Oral petechial lesions.

B Thrombocytopenia in AIDS may be due to a number of causes:
secondary to drugs—AZT, gancyclovir,
infection causing bone marrow suppression, e.g. *Mycobacterium avium intracellulare*,
malignant bone marrow infiltration, e.g. secondary to lymphoma,
autoimmune—ITP secondary to HIV disease.

Answer 126

A Pre-tibial myxoedema.

B Grave's disease.

The typical red/brown thickening of the pretibial skin is associated with Grave's disease, which may have ophthalmic manifestations, such as proptosis (which may be unilateral as in this case), chemosis and ophthalmoplegia.

Question 127

A What condition is shown?

B What are its associations?

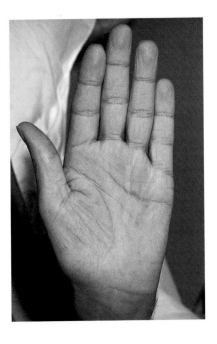

Question 128
These skin lesions have been present for many years in an otherwise well man. What skin condition is shown?

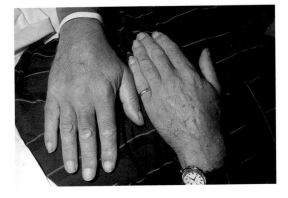

Answer 127

A Palmar erythema.

B Cirrhosis of the liver.
  Rheumatoid arthritis.
  Eczema.
  Psoriasis.
  Diabetes mellitus.

Answer 128

Pustular psoriasis.

This variant of psoriasis affects the palms and the soles with well-demarcated scaling, erythema and sterile pustule formation as the most characteristic feature. There is scaling best demonstrated over the second and third fingers. Although palmar pustular psoriasis is commoner, the dorsum of the hand may also be involved, as in this case.

Question 129
The patient shown here presented with a peripheral neuropathy.

A What lesion is shown?

B What is the underlying condition?

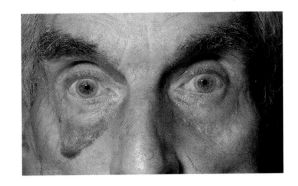

Question 130

A What condition is shown?

B What are its associations?

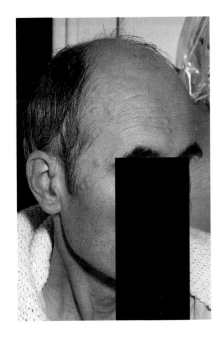

Answer 129

A Periscopic ecchymosis/purpura (an incidental arcus is also present).

B AL amyloidosis.

AL amyloidosis is amyloid of monoclonal immunocytic origin, associated with myeloma and occasionally benign monoclonal gammopathy. The features of this condition include neuropathy, restrictive cardiomyopathy, arthropathy, macroglossia, periorbitol eccymoses and facial purpura.

Answer 130

A Molluscum contagiosum.

B HIV disease.
   idiopathic.

The pearly umbilicated papules of this condition often occur at the margin of the eyelids, and are caused by a pox virus. The lesions are contagious and venereal spread is possible.

Question 131

The 78-year-old male shown here presented with weight loss and haemoptysis. He had been treated for tuberculosis 60 years earlier.

What is the likely cause of his current problems?

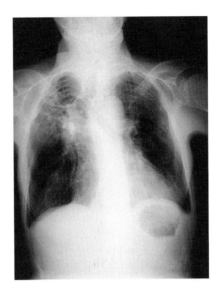

Question 132

The 48-year-old male shown here presented with shortness of breath on exertion and orthopnoea. He was in atrial fibrillation.

A What abnormality is shown?

B What is the underlying diagnosis?

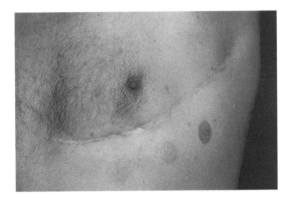

Answer 131

Bronchial carcinoma at the right upper lobe of the lung with old fibrotic changes from tuberculosis (note the shifted trachea).

Reactivation of tuberculosis.

Answer 132

A Thoracotomy scar.

The round red lesion seen to the right of the scar is an artefact of the suction applied to the skin from a single ECG electrode at V4 (seen to a lesser extent at V3).

B Mitral stenosis.

Closed mitral valvotomy is performed via a left thoracotomy. It was a technique used in younger patients with mobile noncalcified valves and no evidence of mitral incompetence. The benefit often lasted for as much as 10–15 years. It is now possible to offer mitral balloon valvuloplasty to patients with such valve characteristics.

Question 133

This 72-year-old ex-shipbuilder presented with shortness of breath and weight loss.

A What is the investigation shown?

B What significant abnormalities are shown?

B What is the likely underlying diagnosis?

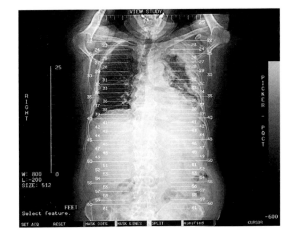

Question 134

This 47-year-old alcoholic subject presented in a confused state. What abnormalities are shown in the abdominal radiograph?

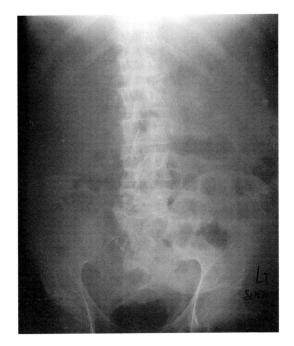

Answer 133

A CT scanogram.

B Pleural thickening left lung.
Left lower lobe consolidation (note air bronchogram).
Enlarged liver.

C Mesothelioma.

Answer 134
Migration of bowel loops to centre of abdomen and ground glass opacification of flanks and pelvis, suggestive of ascites.

Question 135

This 32-year-old was on long-term treatment for a skin disorder.

A What lesion is shown?

B What is the likely underlying diagnosis?

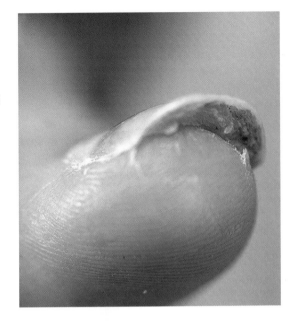

Question 136

The 70-year-old male shown here was under long-term follow-up for coeliac disease. He presented on this occasion with a six-month history of gradually increasing shortness of breath. On examination he was noted to have clubbed fingers.

A What is the likely diagnosis?

B How would you confirm this?

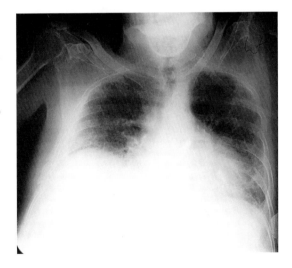

Answer 135

A Subungual hyperkeratosis.

B Psoriasis.

Answer 136

A Cryptogenic fibrosing alveolitis.

B CT scan of the lung.
Bronchoscopy with transbronchial biopsy (bronchoalveolar lavage shows increased neutrophils).
Respiratory lung function tests confirm a restrictive picture with FEV1/FVC > 75%.

The history of coeliac disease with shortness of breath and clubbing is suggestive of the development of cryptogenic fibrosing alveolitis. This is a rare disorder of unknown aetiology that presents in late middle age with shortness of breath, cyanosis and clubbing in two thirds of patients. Bilateral diffuse lung fibrosis occurs often leading to pulmonary hypertension and cor pulmonale. This chest radiograph shows evidence of bilateral reticulonodular shadowing and decreased lung volume. Cryptogenic fibrosing alveolitis is also associated with ulcerative colitis, renal tubular acidosis, ankylosing spondylitis and chronic active hepatitis.

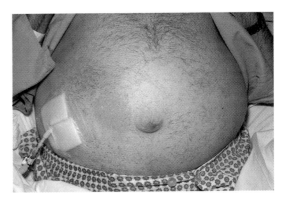

Question 137

This 55-year-old smoker presented with a history of haemoptysis, shortness of breath, weight loss and abdominal distension.

A What abnormalities are shown?

B What is the likely cause of his problems?

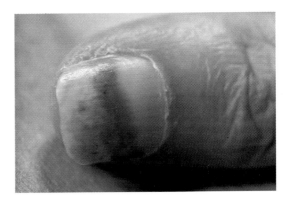

Question 138

A What nail change is shown above?

B What disorders is it associated with?

Answer 137

A Abdominal distension due to ascites.
Umbilical hernia.
Peritoneal drain.

B Bronchial carcinoma with peritoneal and liver metastases leading to ascites.

Answer 138

A Onycholysis: separation of the nail plate from the nail bed.

B Psoriasis, fungal infection, drug eruption, Raynaud's syndrome, trauma, thyrotoxicosis.

Question 139
This 86-year-old male was being ventilated in the intensive care unit after cardiac arrest. His blood gases deteriorated markedly overnight, requiring an emergency procedure.

A What procedure has been carried out?

B What was the cause of his respiratory deterioration?

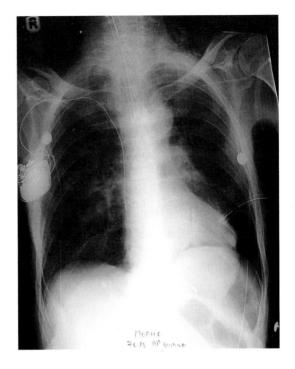

Question 140
The 72-year-old smoker shown here was under review for osteoarthritis in a rheumatology outpatient clinic. The pain in his right shoulder had increased markedly over the previous month.

A What abnormality is shown?

B What is the likely cause?

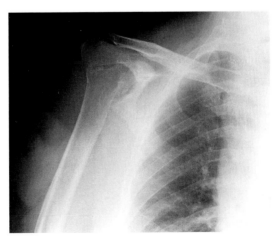

Answer 139

A Chest drain insertion left mid-axillary region.

B Pneumothorax.

Answer 140

A Destruction of the right humeral head.

B Metastatic spread from underlying lung cancer.

Question 141

The CT brain scan shown was taken three months after the patient presented with collapse.

What defect is shown?

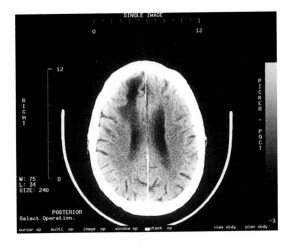

Question 142

The male shown here presented with a flare-up of pain in his foot.

A What abnormality is shown?

B How would you treat him?

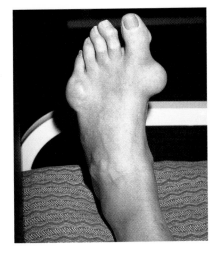

Answer 141

Low attenuation area, right frontal lobe, consistent with resolving infarct (ischaemic or haemorrhagic).

Haemorrhagic strokes initially present as high attenuation areas on contrast-enhanced CT scans. After a two-week period, however, the lesion may become low attenuation, and then become indistinguishable from an ischaemic stroke.

Answer 142

A Tophaceous gout affecting 1st and 5th metatarsophalangeal joints.

B Initially a nonsteroidal anti-inflammatory drug or colchicine should be used to treat the acute attack. After at least four weeks, prophylaxis can be added with either allopurinol (a xanthine oxidase inhibitor) or probenicid (a uricosuric agent) to reduce plasma uric acid levels. Prophylaxis can be continued for life.

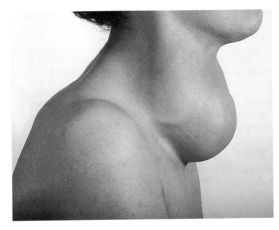

Question 143

This 19-year-old female presented with a chronic neck swelling and deafness.

A What abnormality is shown?

B What is the likely underlying cause?

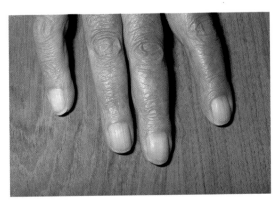

Question 144

What abnormality is shown in this 46-year-old alcoholic?

Answer 143

A Large thyroid goitre.

B Pendred's syndrome.

This chronic presentation would be consistent with an enzyme defect (e.g. Pendred's syndrome) or iodine deficiency. Pendred's syndrome is an autosomal recessive disorder of thyroid hormone synthesis presenting with congenital nerve deafness and a goitre. The biochemical defect in this case is in the generation of peroxidase activity essential for the conversion of iodide to iodine prior to incorporation into the tyrosine residues of thyroglobulin. Thyroid function tests are usually normal (mild hypothyroidism occasionally occurring), a perchlorate discharge test being diagnostic.

Answer 144
Leuconychia.

This condition can be associated with hypoalbuminaemia, in this case secondary to chronic liver disease.

Question 145

The drainage bag in the slide shown here is connected to a chest drain.

A What substance is being drained?

B Give a differential diagnosis for the underlying cause.

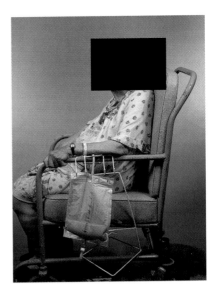

Question 146

What skin condition is shown?

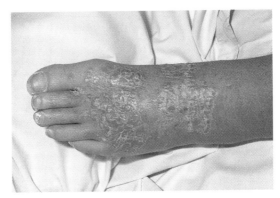

Answer 145

A Chyle.

B Trauma to thoracic duct/ intrathoracic malignancy involving the thoracic duct or subclavian artery/ filarial infection/ lymphangiomyomatosis.

The subdiaphragmatic and left-sided thoracic lymph drains into the thoracic duct. Damage to this structure leads to accumulation of lymph in the pleural space, i.e. a chylothorax. Note that long-standing pleural effusions, e.g. due to tuberculosis and malignancy, may also appear white after time due to the degeneration of cells into cholesterol (pseudochylous) or fat globules (chyliform).

Answer 146

Plaque psoriasis.

Typically salmon pink, well-demarcated plaques with silver scaling are shown. These commonly affect the extensor surfaces of the limbs and are accompanied by arthropathy in 8–10% of those with the condition. Onycholysis can be seen on the third toenail.

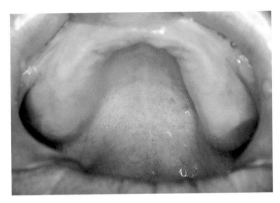

Question 147

This 40-year-old male presented with orthopnoea and shortness of breath on exertion. He was noted to have severe aortic regurgitation on echocardiography.

A What abnormality is shown above?

B What is the likely underlying disorder?

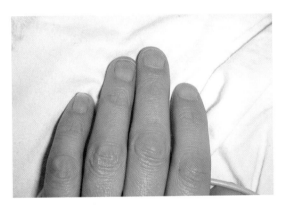

Question 148

A What abnormality is shown in the above slide?

B What is the likely underlying cause?

Answer 147

A High arched palate.

B Marfan's syndrome.

Marfan's syndrome is an autosomal dominant disorder characterized by major and minor phenotypic criteria.

MAJOR
> *Cardiac*
> Mitral valve prolapse with mitral incompetence,
> dilated aortic root with aortic regurgitation,
> dissecting ascending aortic aneurysm.
> *Eye*
> Upward lens dislocation (note that homocystinuria, which may be phenotypically similar to Marfan's, has a downward lens dislocation)

MINOR
> Isolated mitral incompetence,
> high arched palate,
> arachnodactyly,
> joint hypermobility,
> arm span greater than height,
> scoliosis,
> myopia.

Answer 148

A Half and half nails (distal portion brown and proximal portion pale).

B Chronic renal impairment.

Question 149

A What abnormalities are shown in the radiograph?

B What is the likely underlying cause?

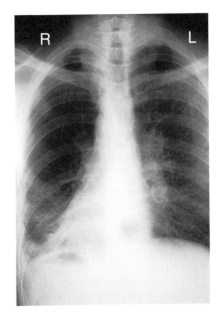

Question 150

This long-standing diabetic patient had this fundal photograph taken at his annual assessment for diabetic retinopathy.

A What does it show?

B What is the most important investigation required?

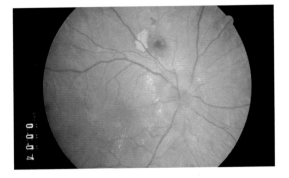

Answer 149

A Dextrocardia.
Situs inversus—gastric bubble on the right-hand side.
Bronchiectasis.
Pulmonary artery enlargement (L > R).

B Kartagener's syndrome.

Bronchiectatic change in this radiograph is suggested by streaky shadows at the left base and multiple thickened end-on bronchi at both bases. The association of bronchiectasis with situs inversus, infertility and chronic sinusitis, is suggestive of Kartagener's syndrome. This has been shown to be related to defects of the dynein arms and radial spokes of the ciliary motor.

Other causes of bronchiectasis may be divided into congenital and acquired:

CONGENITAL
Kartagener's syndrome,
Williams–Campbell syndrome.
ACQUIRED
Post-bronchitis/bronchiolitis,
measles/whooping cough,
cystic fibrosis,
hypogammaglobulinaemia,
lung collapse with infection, e.g. secondary to foreign body inhalation,
bronchial obstruction.

Answer 150

A Dot and blot haemorrhages and hard exudates, i.e. background diabetic retinopathy.
Unexpected papilloedema suggesting raised intracranial pressure.

B CT scan brain.

Question 151

The 25-year-old shown here presented with collapse secondary to subarachnoid haemorrhage. His general practitioner had requested this chest radiograph a year earlier, when the subject had presented with a fever and cough.

A What salient abnormalities are seen on the radiograph above?

B What is the likely underlying condition?

C Give three further complications of this condition.

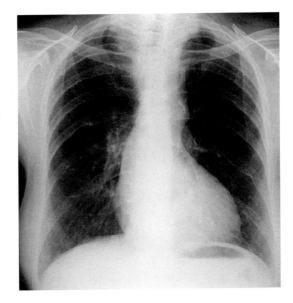

Question 152

A 40-year-old male presented with chest pain and the chest radiograph shown here.

What is the probable diagnosis and which investigation would confirm this?

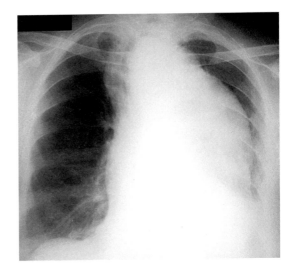

Answer 151

A Rib notching affecting inferior aspects of ribs 3–8 (Dock's sign).

B Coarctation of the aorta.

C Refractory hypertension.
Aortic dissection or rupture.
Endarteritis at the site of the coarctation.

Coarctation of the aorta may lead to refractory hypertension, presenting in this case with a subarachnoid bleed. Rib notching is due to collateralization between the internal mammary and inferior epigastric arteries; it may also be seen in neurofibromatosis.

Answer 152
Widened mediastinum due to ruptured aortic aneurysm.

Investigations: trans-oesophageal echocardiography, MRI or CT scanning.

Question 153

A 30-year-old female presented with a facial rash after a holiday to Marbella. She has a three-month history of joint aches. Give the likeliest diagnosis.

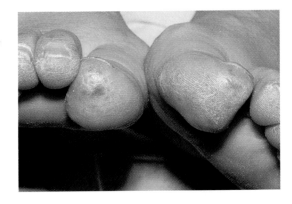

Question 154

This 70-year-old Caucasian female presented with 'pain in her bones'. What is the diagnosis?

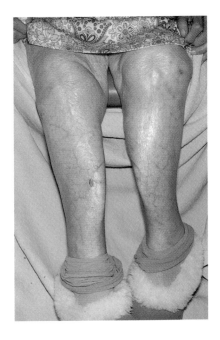

Answer 153

Systemic lupus erythematous.

The slide shows vasculitic lesions of the toes. The photosensitive butterfly facial rash, age and sex of the patient, and the presence of joint pains and vasculitis all suggest SLE.

Answer 154

Sabre tibia secondary to Paget's disease.

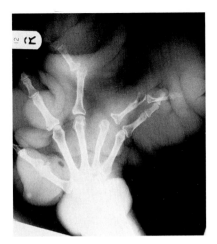

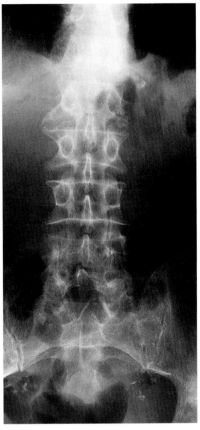

Question 155

The patient shown here has come from a large family cohort with similar deformities.

What is the likely underlying diagnosis?

Question 156

A What is the diagnosis?

B Give the likeliest cause in this 70-year-old male.

Answer 155

This radiograph shows a plexiform neuroma of the hand, otherwise known as elephantiasis neuromatosa, as seen in Von Recklinghausen's disease.

Answer 156

A Destruction of the right pedicle and body of L4 (loss of 'winking owl' appearance).

B Metastatic bone destruction.

Question 157
What is the diagnosis in this 20-year-old male?

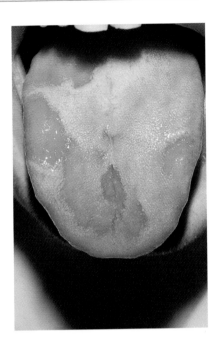

Question 158
This slide shows two pathological processes affecting the nail. Give each of these a differential diagnosis.

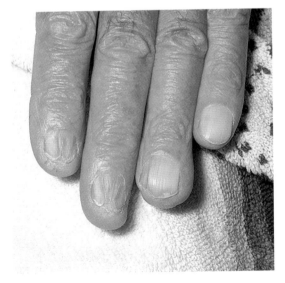

Answer 157

Geographical tongue.

Otherwise known as erythema migrans, this condition is due to loss of papillae, which on regrowth appear to migrate across the surface of the tongue.

Answer 158

Nail fold dystrophy (trauma/ habit tic).

Leuconychia (low protein state in, e.g., nephrotic syndrome/ intestinal malabsorption/ chronic liver disease).

Question 159

A Describe the changes seen here in the fundus.

B What would you expect to find on clinical examination?

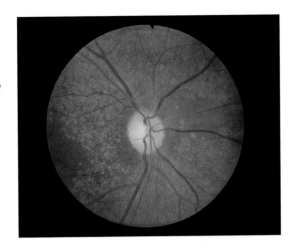

Question 160

What is the abnormality on this chest radiograph?

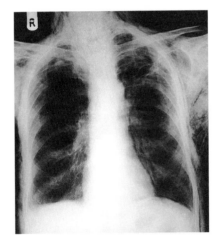

Answer 159

A Optic atrophy with drusen. Drusen are a normal variant.

B Relative afferent pupillary defect on swinging light test (Marcus–Gunn pupil).
Decreased performance on Ischiara charts.
Reduced visual acuity on Snellen chart.

Answer 160

Surgical emphysema with air in the soft tissues of the neck. The cause in this case was a left bronchopleural fistula.

Question 161

This 70-year-old male was on long-term iron treatment.

A What lesion is shown?

B What is the likely underlying condition?

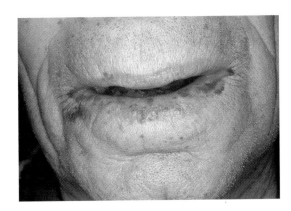

Question 162

This 26-year-old female presented with headache and a rash. She was a frequent attendee at hospital casualty departments. What condition is shown?

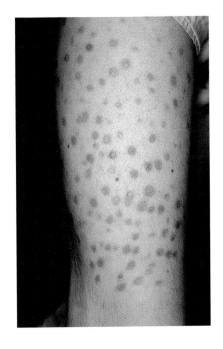

Answer 161

A Multiple telangiectasia around the lips.

B Osler–Weber–Rendu syndrome (hereditary haemorrhagic telangiectasia).

This autosomal dominant condition leads to skin and mucosal telangiectasia. It often presents with iron deficiency anaemia secondary to occult gastro-intestinal bleeding.

Answer 162
Dermatitis artefacta.

These symmetrical lesions were created using a cigarette stub. Patients such as the subject shown often have a long history of personality disorder.

Question 163
This 30-year-old woman presented with abdominal pain. What sign is shown? What is the mechanism?

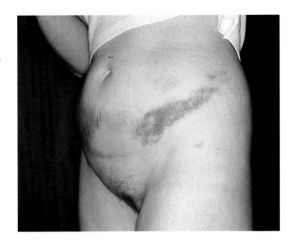

Question 164
This 53-year-old man with myeloma presented with severe shortness of breath.

What abnormalities are shown on the chest radiograph?

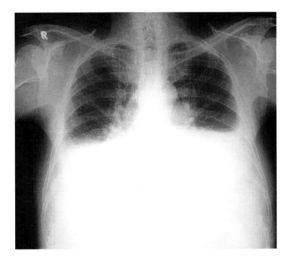

Answer 163
Grey Turner's sign: abdominal wall ecchymoses in the flanks seen in acute pancreatitis. Proteases and lipases leak into the abdomen and cause proteolysis and lipolysis. Cullen's sign may also occur (periumbilical abdominal wall eccymoses).

Answer 164
Bilateral pleural effusions.

Question 165

This 25-year-old smoker presented with severe foot pain.

A What does this photograph of his foot demonstrate?

B What is the underlying diagnosis?

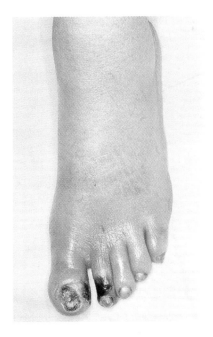

Answer 165

A Gangrene of the first and second toe; shiny and hairless skin.

B Buerger's disease (thromboangiitis obliterans).

Index